# High-Energy, Nutrient-Dense Emergency Relief Food Product

Subcommittee on Technical Specifications for a
High-Energy Emergency Relief Ration

Committee on Military Nutrition Research

Food and Nutrition Board

INSTITUTE OF MEDICINE

NATIONAL ACADEMY PRESS
Washington, D.C.

**NATIONAL ACADEMY PRESS • 2101 Constitution Avenue, N.W. • Washington, DC 20418**

NOTICE: The project that is the subject of this report was approved by the Governing Board of the National Research Council, whose members are drawn from the councils of the National Academy of Sciences, the National Academy of Engineering, and the Institute of Medicine. The members of the committee responsible for the report were chosen for their special competences and with regard for appropriate balance.

Support for this project was provided by the U.S. Department of the Army, Army Medical Research and Materiel Command through grant No. DAMD17-99-1-9478. The U.S. Army Medical Research Acquisition Activity, 820 Chandler Street, Fort Detrick, MD 21702-5014, is the awarding and administering acquisition office. The views presented in this publication are those of the Subcommittee on Technical Specifications for a High-Energy Emergency Relief Ration and do not necessarily reflect the position or policy of the government, and no official endorsement should be inferred.

International Standard Book Number: 0-309-08315-X
Library of Congress Control Number: 2002101391

Additional copies of this report are available for sale from the National Academy Press, 2101 Constitution Avenue, N.W., Box 285, Washington, D.C. 20055. Call (800) 624-6242 or (202) 334-3313 (in the Washington metropolitan area), or visit the NAP's home page at **www.nap.edu.** The full text of this report is available at **www.nap.edu.**

For more information about the Institute of Medicine, visit the IOM home page at: **www.iom.edu.**



Printed in the United States of America.

The serpent has been a symbol of long life, healing, and knowledge among almost all cultures and religions since the beginning of recorded history. The serpent adopted as a logotype by the Institute of Medicine is a relief carving from ancient Greece, now held by the Staatliche Museen in Berlin.

Cover photo courtesy of Marjatta Tolvanen.

*"Knowing is not enough; we must apply.
Willing is not enough; we must do."*
—Goethe

INSTITUTE OF MEDICINE

Shaping the Future for Health

# THE NATIONAL ACADEMIES

National Academy of Sciences
National Academy of Engineering
Institute of Medicine
National Research Council

The **National Academy of Sciences** is a private, nonprofit, self-perpetuating society of distinguished scholars engaged in scientific and engineering research, dedicated to the furtherance of science and technology and to their use for the general welfare. Upon the authority of the charter granted to it by the Congress in 1863, the Academy has a mandate that requires it to advise the federal government on scientific and technical matters. Dr. Bruce M. Alberts is president of the National Academy of Sciences.

The **National Academy of Engineering** was established in 1964, under the charter of the National Academy of Sciences, as a parallel organization of outstanding engineers. It is autonomous in its administration and in the selection of its members, sharing with the National Academy of Sciences the responsibility for advising the federal government. The National Academy of Engineering also sponsors engineering programs aimed at meeting national needs, encourages education and research, and recognizes the superior achievements of engineers. Dr. Wm. A. Wulf is president of the National Academy of Engineering.

The **Institute of Medicine** was established in 1970 by the National Academy of Sciences to secure the services of eminent members of appropriate professions in the examination of policy matters pertaining to the health of the public. The Institute acts under the responsibility given to the National Academy of Sciences by its congressional charter to be an adviser to the federal government and, upon its own initiative, to identify issues of medical care, research, and education. Dr. Kenneth I. Shine is president of the Institute of Medicine.

The **National Research Council** was organized by the National Academy of Sciences in 1916 to associate the broad community of science and technology with the Academy's purposes of furthering knowledge and advising the federal government. Functioning in accordance with general policies determined by the Academy, the Council has become the principal operating agency of both the National Academy of Sciences and the National Academy of Engineering in providing services to the government, the public, and the scientific and engineering communities. The Council is administered jointly by both Academies and the Institute of Medicine. Dr. Bruce M. Alberts and Dr. Wm. A. Wulf are chairman and vice chairman, respectively, of the National Research Council.

## SUBCOMMITTEE ON TECHNICAL SPECIFICATIONS FOR A HIGH-ENERGY EMERGENCY RELIEF RATION

**BARRY L. ZOUMAS** (*chair*), Department of Agricultural Economics and Rural Sociology, The Pennsylvania State University, University Park

**LAWRENCE E. ARMSTRONG**, Departments of Kinesiology, Nutritional Sciences, and Physiology and Neurobiology, University of Connecticut, Storrs

**JEFFREY R. BACKSTRAND**, Program in Urban Systems, University of Medicine and Dentistry of New Jersey, Newark

**WANDA L. CHENOWETH**, Department of Food Science and Human Nutrition, Michigan State University, East Lansing

**PAVINEE CHINACHOTI**, Department of Food Science and Nutrition, University of Massachusetts, Amherst

**BARBARA P. KLEIN**, Department of Food Science and Human Nutrition, University of Illinois, Urbana

**HELEN W. LANE**, Advanced Human Support Technologies Program, NASA Johnson Space Center, Houston, Texas

**KENNETH S. MARSH**, Kenneth S. Marsh & Associates, Ltd., Seneca, South Carolina

**MARJATTA TOLVANEN**, Nutrition in Emergencies, UNICEF, New York, New York

*Staff*

**RICARDO MOLINS**, Study Director

**MARY I. POOS**, Senior Program Officer

**LESLIE J. VOGELSANG**, Research Assistant

**TAZIMA L. DAVIS**, Senior Project Assistant

## COMMITTEE ON MILITARY NUTRITION RESEARCH

**JOHN E. VANDERVEEN** (*chair*), San Antonio, Texas
**BRUCE R. BISTRIAN**, Department of Medicine, Beth Israel Deaconess Medical Center, Boston, Massachusetts
**JOHANNA T. DWYER**, Agricultural Research Service, U.S. Department of Agriculture, Washington, D.C.
**JOHN W. ERDMAN, Jr.**, Division of Nutritional Science, University of Illinois at Urbana-Champaign
**HELEN W. LANE**, Advanced Human Support Technologies Program, NASA Johnson Space Center, Houston, Texas
**MELINDA MANORE**, Department of Nutrition and Food Management, Oregon State University, Corvallis
**WILLIAM P. MORGAN**, Sport Psychology Laboratory, University of Wisconsin, Madison
**PATRICK M. O'NEIL**, Weight Management Center, Medical University of South Carolina, Charleston
**ESTHER M. STERNBERG**, Neuroendocrine Immunology and Behavior Section, National Institute of Mental Health, Bethesda, Maryland
**BEVERLY J. TEPPER**, Department of Food Science, Rutgers University, New Brunswick, New Jersey

*U.S. Army Grant Representative*
**LTC KARL E. FRIEDL**, Military Operational Medicine Research Program, U.S. Army Medical Research and Materiel Command, Fort Detrick, Frederick, Maryland

*Staff*
**MARY I. POOS**, Study Director
**LESLIE J. VOGELSANG**, Research Assistant
**TAZIMA A. DAVIS**, Senior Project Assistant

## FOOD AND NUTRITION BOARD

# Acknowledgments

The Subcommittee on Technical Specifications for a High-Energy Emergency Relief Ration thanks all individuals and institutions that contributed information, time, and funds to this report. Special thanks are given to Samuel Kahn, Thomas Marchione, and other personnel of the U.S. Agency for International Development (USAID) and the U.S. Department of Defense, and to USAID consultants Michael Golden, Caroline Grobler-Tanner, and Mary Lung'aho, who contributed valuable written and verbal information to the subcommittee during its open discussions. Especially helpful were the information and experience shared with the subcommittee by the U.S. Department of Defense Combat Feeding Program, Performance Enhancement and Food Safety Team, during its first meeting, graciously hosted by the U.S. Army Soldier Systems Center, Natick, Massachusetts, with a special thanks to Major Maria Bovill, who so capably organized all the meeting logistics for the subcommittee at Natick, including suggesting hotels and restaurants and providing directions from Boston to the Center.

This report has been reviewed in draft form by individuals chosen for their diverse perspectives and technical expertise, in accordance with procedures approved by the NRC's Report Review Committee. The purpose of this independent review is to provide candid and critical comments that will assist the institution in making its published report as sound as possible and to ensure that the report meets institutional standards for objectivity, evidence, and responsiveness to the study charge. The review comments and draft manuscript remain confidential to protect the integrity of the deliberative process. We wish to thank the following individuals for their review of this report:

Lindsay H. Allen, Ph.D., R.D.
E. Wayne Askew, Ph.D.
Johanna Dwyer, D.Sc., R.D.
Theodore Labuza, Ph.D.
John H. Litchfield, Ph.D.
Irwin H. Rosenberg, M.D.

Although the reviewers listed above have provided many constructive comments and suggestions, they were not asked to endorse the conclusions or recommendations nor did they see the final draft of the report before its release. The review of this report was overseen by Barbara Underwood, Ph.D., Scholar-in-Residence, Institute of Medicine. Appointed by the National Research Council and Institute of Medicine, she was responsible for making certain that an independent examination of this report was carried out in accordance with institutional procedures and that all review comments were carefully considered. Responsibility for the final content of this report rests entirely with the authoring committee and the institution.

The subcommittee presents its special appreciation to the Institute of Medicine staff who facilitated the work and the preparation of this report: Ricardo Molins, study director; Mary Poos, study director of the Committee on Military Nutrition Research; Gail Spears, who edited the report; Leslie Vogelsang, research assistant; Tazima Davis, senior project assistant; and Allison Yates, director of the Food and Nutrition Board.

Barry Zoumas, Chair
Subcommittee on Technical Specifications for a High-Energy Emergency Relief Ration

# Contents

# Executive Summary

As the world enters a new millennium, natural disasters and international or internal conflicts continue to displace hundreds of thousands of people. The human and physical needs of disaster and other emergency victims—deprived of or uprooted from their homes, on the road or in crowded camps and exposed to harsh elements—are paramount in efforts to provide a significant measure of relief. In response to the plight of refugees, the United States has provided assistance in many ways to victims of such emergencies the world over, most notably via food programs.

To a large extent, the emergency food relief assistance provided by the U.S. government has been channeled through the U.S. Agency for International Development (USAID) and the Department of Defense (DOD). The bulk of medium- and long-term food relief contributed by USAID has traditionally been in the form of commodity foods. However, USAID and DOD also participate in rapid, short-term food relief operations that require special high-energy, self-contained food products not currently manufactured in the United States. Such products constitute the vanguard of food relief and are designed for use over the normally short period of time needed to establish a more permanent, stable, food-based relief pipeline. Because of legislative restrictions on the use of some federal appropriations, only limited purchases of such products can be made by USAID from food manufacturers outside the United States. The availability of science-based technical specifications for use in calls for bids from U.S. food manufacturers, therefore, is of the essence not only to allow procurement of the most appropriate product, but also to do so in the United States.

## BACKGROUND AND CHARGE TO THE COMMITTEE

The present study was conducted by an ad hoc subcommittee of the Committee on Military Nutrition Research. The Subcommittee on Technical Specifications for a High-Energy Emergency Relief Ration was established by the Food and Nutrition Board of the Institute of Medicine in response to a request from USAID and DOD to develop technical specifications for a product for use in food relief after natural disasters or other emergency situations around the world. The specifications are to be used by both agencies in their calls for bids from U.S. food manufacturers to supply such a product.

The charge to the subcommittee was as follows: Based on information on the nutritional requirements of target populations, food/nutrition specifications, product descriptions of similar rations already in use (e.g., emergency biscuits), and recommendations by refugee nutrition experts, what are the committee's recommendations to these questions:

1. What are the specifications for a cost-effective emergency ration bar for uprooted people in emergency situations that meets all of the following criteria:
   a. satisfies all nutrient requirements for a population of all ages over 6 months
   b. appropriate for use as the sole source of subsistence for up to 15 days
   c. acceptable to people of any ethnic and religious background
   d. can be eaten on the move without preparation steps
   e. can, without significant cost increase, be prepositioned in harsh environments for at least 3 years
   f. can, without significant cost increase, withstand an airdrop without endangering persons on the ground

2. Specifications should include consideration of each of these categories:
   a. *nutritional composition*, including macro- and micronutrient content and water content
   b. *food properties*, including nutrient stability, food consistency, palatability, and organoleptics
   c. *universal acceptance*, especially cultural acceptability to refugees and displaced persons
   d. *configuration*, size, color, and shape
   e. *packaging* for shipping, long-term stability (3 years), stability for airdrop, and ease of use
   f. *feasibility of manufacture*
   g. *commodity cost within limitations of average relief operations*

3. Make recommendations on special circumstances when this ration should and should not be used (and any provisions for simple alternatives or supplements), including:
   a. severely malnourished groups of refugees or liberated prisoners of war who may have specific micronutrient deficiencies or protein deficiency
   b. populations with a high prevalence of disease, such as acquired immune deficiency syndrome or diarrheal diseases
   c. individuals in harsh environmental conditions.

## METHODS

The subcommittee met twice during the study. The first meeting was held at the U.S. Army Soldier Systems Center, Natick, Massachusetts, to allow the subcommittee to benefit from the experience of the DOD Combat Feeding Program, Performance Enhancement and Food Safety Team, and thus gather information on processes, ingredients, and packaging systems used by the U.S. Army in developing products similar to the desired emergency food product (EFP). Also at this meeting, USAID representatives described the agency's worldwide emergency food relief programs, and three USAID consultants discussed two background papers commissioned for this purpose by the agency. Moreover, the consultants contributed invaluable information on field conditions during emergency food relief operations that were taken into consideration by the subcommittee in its deliberations. The second and final subcommittee meeting was held in Washington, D.C.

## REPORT ORGANIZATION

The report contains four chapters. Chapter 1 summarizes the project scope, its rationale, and the background for the need and uses of an EFP. It describes the types of emergencies and populations expected to benefit from such a product, and the special circumstances inherent to food relief operations after natural or man-made disasters, famines, massive displacement of people, and other emergencies that must be considered in defining the nutritional, chemical, and physical characteristics the EFP should have.

Chapter 2 describes the basic assumptions underlying the energy level chosen for the EFP, the calculations of macro- and micronutrient levels, and, in some instances, the recommended origin or modality of the nutrients to be used. The daily energy requirement recommended for planning emergency aid rations by a 1995 IOM report (2,100 kcal/day) was adopted by the subcommittee. Fundamental assumptions made by the subcommittee in determining the nutritional content of the EFP are given in Box ES-1.

Each macro- and micronutrient specification is discussed individually in Chapter 2. However, the subcommittee's recommendation for each is presented

**BOX ES-1** Assumptions Used in Developing the Nutrition Composition of the EFP

- Potable water is provided as a top priority and is available with the EFP.
- Individuals will eat to meet their energy requirements.
- The product is to be consumed by all age groups, except infants less than 6 months of age; thus the product is not to be used in lieu of breast feeding, which is encouraged to at least 1 year of age with complementary use of the EFP after 6 months of age.
- It is not to be used as a therapeutic product and is not appropriate for severely malnourished individuals.
- It may constitute the sole source of food for target recipients for up to 15 days.
- Recipients are likely to be at least mildly malnourished and/or suffer from mild to moderate diarrhea and other debilitating diseases brought about by unsanitary conditions and exacerbated by stress.
- The recipient population may have nutrient needs comparable to well-nourished individuals in spite of smaller body weights due to maintaining muscle and visceral mass at the expense of body fat.
- The product should provide a nutrient density that will meet or exceed the nutrient recommendations as specified by the recommended intakes (IOM, 1997, 1998, 2000, 2001; NRC, 1989) which are designed to meet the needs of almost all individuals in each life stage and gender group (with the exception of infants) without exceeding Tolerable Upper Intake Levels (IOM, 1997, 1998, 2000, 2001).
- Nutrient needs of pregnant and lactating women are not included in the calculations, but it is assumed they will consume more than the daily ration based on individual needs for additional energy beyond the average of 2,100 kcal/day.

in tabular form in Chapter 4 (as Table 4-1) for ease of use by the agencies and potential manufacturers.

Chapter 3 discusses the preservation, processing, and packaging techniques that manufacturers should use in preparing the EFP so that it will attain the required stability under the expected conditions of delivery and use. These conditions might include extreme temperatures, rough handling, improvised storage, and the possible need to airdrop the product from low altitude. The recommendations from Chapter 3 are presented in the form of a performance specification for use by the agencies in preparing a call for bids in Chapter 4. The subcommittee views the technical specifications recommended in this report as optimal, but recognizes that the sponsoring agencies may be forced to consider developing EFPs prepared and packaged in less desirable ways if cost becomes the primary consideration.

## RECOMMENDATIONS

There are five characteristics critical to development of a successful EFP. These are listed in order of importance. The EFP must be:

1. Safe
2. Palatable
3. Easy to deliver
4. Easy to use
5. Nutritionally complete.

In terms of decisions in the development of a prototype, this order of importance of the EFP should guide decisions about trade-offs between competing characteristics. In addition, it is recognized that the EFP must meet economical considerations; although considered in developing the specifications, it was beyond the scope of this report to weigh technical and nutritional advantages versus cost in a cost–benefit analysis. In addition to the recommended levels of each macro- and micronutrient presented in Table ES-1, the following recommendations are made:

- **Microbiological stability.** Preservation techniques that include combinations of low water activity values and some preservative(s) are the best approach to achieve microbiological stability of the EFP.
- **Chemical stability and nutrient retention.** A water activity level lower than 0.4 in the EFP is necessary to ensure protection against nutrient degradation. Microencapsulation of selected components and nutrients, particularly vitamin E together with highly unsaturated lipids, ascorbic acid, and iron (as FeNa EDTA), and other minerals is essential to minimize adverse lipid oxidation and nutrient losses. Antioxidants could be used in combination with microencapsulation depending on the ingredients used to prepare the EFP.
- **Flavor and color.** Based on anecdotal information, is suggested that only a sweet flavor and natural colors be used. The product, if dispersed in water, must not resemble milk. However, potential manufacturers should be encouraged to propose other flavors for the EFP, but these flavors should be tested for acceptability as described below.
- **Ingredients.** The ingredients used to prepare the EFP must provide the nutritional profile and other characteristics defined in the specifications. However, because the product will be distributed among multiple ethnic and cultural groups, alcohol or animal products other than milk may not be used. Use of milk solids must be limited so that lactose levels are not in excess of amounts known to be tolerated by individuals who are lactose maldigestors. Foods containing known allergens, such as peanuts, should be avoided. Some

**TABLE ES-1** Nutritional Content of the Emergency Relief Food Product (EFP)[a]

| Nutrient | Limiting Group | Minimum Required Nutrient Density per 1,000 kcal[a] | Amount per Single (233 kcal; 50g) EFP Bar |
|---|---|---|---|
| Fat | N/A | | 9–12 g |
| Protein[b] | 51+ yr, men | | 7.9 g |
| Carbohydrate | N/A | | 23–35 g |
| Sodium[c] | 2–5 yr, children | 1.3 g | 300 mg |
| Potassium[c] | 2–5 yr, children | 1.7 g | 396 mg |
| Chloride[c] | 2–5 yr, children | 2.0 g | 466 mg |
| Calcium | 9–13 yr, children | 768 mg | 180 mg |
| Phosphorus | 9–13 yr, children | 740 mg | 172 mg |
| Magnesium | 14–18 yr, boys | 190 mg | 45 mg |
| Chromium | — | 13 μg[d] | 3 μg |
| Copper | 51+ yr, women | 560 μg[d] | 131 μg |
| Iodine | 1–3 yr, children | 105 μg | 25 μg |
| Iron[e] | 19–50 yr, women | 16 mg[d] | 3.8 mg |
| Manganese | 1–3 yr, children | 1.4 mg | 0.33 mg |
| Selenium | 14–18 yr, girls | 28 μg | 6.5 μg |
| Zinc | 14–18 yr, boys | 10.5 mg[d] | 2.4 mg |
| Vitamin A | 14–18 yr, boys | 500 μg[d] | 117 μg |
| Vitamin D | 51–70 yr, women | 5.2 μg[d] | 1.2 μg |
| Vitamin E | 14–18 yr, girls | 16 mg[d] | 2.2 mg |
| Vitamin K | 19–50 yr, men | 60 μg | 14 μg |
| Vitamin C | 51+ yr, men | 100 mg[d] | 11.1 mg |
| Thiamin | 1–3 yr, children | 1.2 mg[d] | 0.28 mg |
| Riboflavin | 14–18 yr, boys | 1.2 mg[d] | 0.28 mg |
| Niacin | 14–18 yr, boys | 11.2 mg NE[d] | 2.6 mg NE |
| Vitamin $B_6$ | 51+ yr, women | 1.2 mg[d] | 0.28 mg[e] |
| Folate[f] | 14–18 yr, girls | 310 μg DFE[d] | 72 μg DFE |
| Vitamin $B_{12}$ | 14–18 yr, girls | 12 μg[d] | 2.8 μg |
| Pantothenic acid | 14–18 yr, girls | 3.9 mg[d] | 0.9 mg |
| Biotin | 51+, women | 24 μg[d] | 5.6 μg |
| Choline | 51+, men | 366 mg[d] | 85 mg |

[a] Ration set at 2,100 kcal/d (IOM, 1995).
[b] From NRC (1989); based on reference weights from IOM (1997) and estimated energy expenditure from Table 2-3.
[c] Values based on estimated requirements or desirable intakes (NRC, 1989).
[d] Adjusted from baseline nutrient density value; see text for explanation.
[e] Based on 10% iron bioavailability.
[f] If folate is provided as synthetic folate, which is more readily absorbed, these numbers should be divided by 1.6.
SOURCE: IOM (1997, 1998, 2000, 2001).

recommended ingredients are the following in order to provide nutrients as specified (see Table ES-1):

- cereal base: wheat flour, corn, oat flakes or flour, rice flour
- protein: soy products, such as concentrates or isolates; milk solids, casein, or derivatives; mixture of cereal base and protein must have a Protein Digestibility-Corrected Amino Acid Score ≥ 1.0
- lipid sources: partially hydrogenated soybean or cottonseed oil, flaxseed oil (source of omega-3 fatty acids), canola oil, sunflower oil
- sugars: sucrose, glucose, high-fructose corn syrup, maltodextrins
- baking and leavening agents, if needed
- vitamin and mineral premix as specified in the nutrient profile.

• **Testing prototypes for acceptability.** All EFP prototypes should be tested for acceptability under conditions similar to those used by the U.S. Army for General Purpose Survival Packets and Meal Ready-to-Eat, Individual. The suggestion made by the U.S. Army to use its facilities at various overseas locations for testing the EFP among local populations, so that its acceptability by populations having diverse ethnic and cultural backgrounds can be established, is heartily endorsed.

• **Packaging.** All packaging components used in the EFP must be capable of withstanding a wide range of temperatures and other physical abuse. Separate or additional packaging may be necessary for EFP airdrop operations. Pulp-based material with a moisture barrier coating should be used for the EFP primary packaging. A pouch constructed of a trilaminate consisting inside out of polyolefin, aluminum foil, and polyester or nylon should be the secondary packaging to keep oxygen at less than 2 percent throughout the 3-year shelf life of the product. Optional presentations of the EFP other than that for airdrop configuration could include a reusable, semi-rigid polyolefin, multi-ration container appropriately designed to allow secondary uses such as storage or water transport. Alternatively, a metal outer package, such as a tinplate box with an easy-to-remove cover, would be of great value to recipients during emergencies.

• **Product configuration.** The recommended 2,100-kcal/day energy level should be provided by an EFP weighing approximately 450 g. This ration should be configured as nine equal portions having the shape of bars, each scored across the width of the bar to provide two 116-kcal portions upon breaking it. A daily supply of nine bars should be packaged under a nitrogen flush or vacuum into one trilaminate pouch to provide the barrier against oxygen and moisture needed for extended shelf life. Five daily rations should be packaged into a single bundle so that 5-days worth of food for a single individual or a 1-day feeding of a five-member family may be distributed as a unit. Eight bundles of five EFPs each should be placed into a shipping container of corrugated construction or constructed of metal, so that they can be recycled for use as storage or water containers. Shippers would be assembled onto a pallet for transport.

- **Production methods.** The EFP must be prepared using Good Manufacturing Practices and all sanitary regulations and practices applicable to ready-to-eat food products.

- **Testing for quality assurance and control.** Testing of the EFP must be conducted throughout the expected shelf life of the product and under conditions of delivery and storage simulating actual use, to ascertain the initial content and stability of nutrients throughout the expected 3-year shelf life. Standard methodologies for determining vitamin and mineral content of the EFP should be used, and appropriate procedures, such as those used for nutritional labeling, must be applied.

## REFERENCES

IOM (Institute of Medicine). 1995. *Estimated Mean per Capita Energy Requirements for Planning Emergency Food Aid Rations*. Washington, DC: National Academy Press.

IOM. 1997. *Dietary Reference Intakes for Calcium, Phosphorus, Magnesium, Vitamin D, and Fluoride*. Washington, DC: National Academy Press.

IOM. 1998. *Dietary Reference Intakes for Thiamin, Riboflavin, Niacin, Vitamin* $B_6$*, Folate, Vitamin* $B_{12}$*, Pantothenic Acid, Biotin, and Choline*. Washington, DC: National Academy Press.

IOM. 2000. *Dietary Reference Intakes for Vitamin C, Vitamin E, Selenium, and Carotenoids*. Washington, DC: National Academy Press.

IOM. 2001. *Dietary Reference Intakes for Vitamin A, Vitamin K, Arsenic, Boron, Chromium, Copper, Iodine, Iron, Manganese, Molybdenum, Nickel, Silicon, Vanadium, and Zinc*. Washington, DC: National Academy Press.

NRC (National Research Council). 1989. *Recommended Dietary Allowances*. 10th ed. Washington, DC: National Academy Press.

# 1
# Introduction

## PROJECT DESCRIPTION AND SCOPE

The Subcommittee on Technical Specifications for a High-Energy Emergency Relief Ration was established by the Food and Nutrition Board, Institute of Medicine (IOM) of The National Academies under the oversight of the standing Committee on Military Nutrition Research. The subcommittee was formed to address a request from the U.S. Agency for International Development (USAID) of the Department of State and the Department of Defense (DOD). These agencies asked IOM to develop technical specifications to be used in their solicitation of bids from the U.S. food industry for the production of a high-energy, nutrient-dense emergency relief food product (EFP). The scope of the subcommittee's task centered on defining the specifications of an EFP that would satisfy the nutritional requirements of populations of all ages above 6 months, be appropriate for use as the sole source of subsistence for up to 15 days, be acceptable to a wide spectrum of cultures and ethnic and religious backgrounds, be eaten on the move without need for preparation, be stable for at least 3 years, and be amenable to land or air delivery.

The specifications requested for an EFP encompassed the following: nutritional composition, including water and macro- and micronutrient content; food properties related to stability, consistency, and sensory properties and acceptability; product configuration, size, color, shape, and primary and secondary packaging for long-term prepositioning under severe environmental conditions and for land or air delivery; feasibility of manufacture; quality assurance and control parameters; and estimated cost.

In addition, the subcommittee was asked to make recommendations on when the EFP should and should not be used. Finally, it was requested that the report present all relevant product characteristics and other processing and quality control parameters in performance specification format.

## ORIGIN OF THE STUDY

Feeding refugees or disaster victims depends on being able to deliver a nutritionally appropriate diet quickly and at low cost. USAID, through its recently created Democracy, Conflict and Humanitarian Assistance Bureau (which includes the former Bureau for Humanitarian Response), assists foreign countries in famine and disaster relief by providing food rations for distribution. Similar humanitarian aid is provided by DOD in emergency situations. This food relief is often the only source of food available to affected individuals during the initial period after such natural disasters as hurricanes or earthquakes, or during emergencies such as evacuations or fleeing from combat zones.

The energy value, nutritional composition, and sensory appeal of emergency food rations are of utmost importance in meeting the nutritional needs of recipients. In general, emergency food relief has traditionally relied on distribution of bulk food such as grains or corn- or wheat-based mixes that require preparation prior to consumption. The aim of the present study, in contrast, is to provide specifications for a stand-alone product that can be delivered and used as a sole source of food while a more permanent, stable food relief system is established. It is possible that the EFP could be used later in circumstances other than emergencies as a supplemental source of nutrients to more traditional diets.

In addition to the overriding importance of having a food ration that provides the required energy level, protein, vitamins, minerals, and other essential nutrients, sensory appeal is an important factor to be considered when developing formulations that may be acceptable to a wide spectrum of cultures. Maintaining quality and appropriate package design, in turn, are critical to meeting the food relief objective because the rations must be able to endure very harsh conditions during handling and storage with minimal nutrient losses. The size and type of packaging has also proven to be important to avoid diversion of the EFPs to military use during emergencies involving civilian populations and combatants. Because of logistic problems during many emergencies, it is also essential that packaging of the EFPs be specially designed to withstand an airdrop without being destroyed or harming recipients on the ground.

Although the United States is a major contributor to global food relief, U.S. companies do not currently manufacture the type of food products necessary for the initial stages of emergency food relief. As a result, and because USAID is required to purchase only U.S. products with Public Law (P.L.) 480 funds, purchases of such products from European manufacturers (see Chapter 3) can only be made by USAID using other limited funds. The availability of specifications for use in solicitations of bids from the U.S. food industry, therefore, will allow not only procurement of the most appropriate product, but also one that is manufactured within the United States.

## THE NEED FOR AND USES OF A HIGH-ENERGY, NUTRIENT-DENSE EMERGENCY RELIEF FOOD PRODUCT

### Emergencies Requiring Relief Operations

Disasters requiring food relief operations include natural disasters, man-made disasters, and complex humanitarian emergencies. Natural disasters are those caused by fire, flood, drought, earthquake, and disease outbreak, whereas man-made disasters are caused by human error, as in industrial accidents. Complex humanitarian emergencies are usually the result of or complicated by armed conflict, genocide, or rural famines, and tend to cause massive population displacements aggravated by the lack or collapse of basic services (Keely et al., 2001). The extent and level of complexity of these emergencies may be further compounded by natural weather phenomena such as droughts or by unique circumstances such as the presence of large populations of prisoners of war. Some 30 complex humanitarian emergencies existed worldwide at the end of 1999 (Keely et al., 2001).

Natural disasters and their impact on people are on the increase, according to U.S. relief organizations. Causes identified by USAID (2001a) include the continuous degradation of natural environments that magnify the impact of natural events, and population increases in coastal areas and other regions exposed to floods, eruptions, landslides, and other geological or meteorological threats (USAID, 2001b). Examples of environmental degradation contributing to natural disasters are destruction of forests, desertification, and overall climate change. The number of natural disasters in the 1990s—designated by the United Nations General Assembly in its resolution 44/236 as the International Decade for Natural Disaster Reduction—tripled that seen in the 1960s. The Office of the U.N. Emergency Relief Coordinator estimated that from 1970 to 1990 some 800 million people were affected by natural disasters, including more than 3 million deaths, with cumulative economic losses in the order of $30 to $50 billion per year (UNEP, 1992).

According to USAID, almost 2 billion people were affected by natural disasters globally during the 1990s (USAID, 2001b). In 1999 alone, 212 million people were affected by hurricanes, typhoons, earthquakes, and floods that required immediate response from national and international relief organizations. This number did not include the hundreds of millions of people affected by droughts and their sequel of famines, many of whom abandoned their homes, villages, and regions in search of food for survival, nor the some 35 million people uprooted by 25 armed conflicts in 27 countries that year. Among the latter, 21 million were classified as internally displaced persons (IDPs), while the other 14 million, having crossed international boundaries, were classified as refugees (Crisp, 2000; USCR, 2000). Statistics from the office of the United Nations High Commissioner for Refugees (UNCHR) for 2000 list 21 million people as "refugees and others of concern"; 12 million of these were refugees (UNHCR, 2001).

Emergency relief is provided by the United States and other donors in regions of the world where natural disasters occur and the affected country does not have the capacity to cope with destruction of the public service infrastructure. It is also provided when complex humanitarian emergencies induce massive population displacements through or into areas where public services are nonexistent or insufficient (Keely et al., 2001). Many situations requiring emergency relief arise in the least developed, poorest areas of the world, where human populations are frequently afflicted with chronic malnutrition and various debilitating diseases such as dysentery and malaria (de Onis, 2000; Snow et al., 1999). The threat to life as well as the psychological distress associated with the loss of homes and livelihoods, and sometimes the horrors of combat situations, are other important contributing factors to the overall weakness and poor physical state of populations in need of emergency relief (Burkholder et al., 2001). These often result in high mortality rates, particularly among children in developing countries and the elderly in more developed areas (Keely et al., 2001).

Although it has been said that the only common denominator in emergencies requiring relief is that they are all unique and different, the need for foods with acceptable quality attributes and in quantities appropriate to sustain those affected is also common to all, as is the need to deliver such food promptly and at low cost. It is generally agreed among relief organizations that the quality of food relief provided to affected individuals during the initial stages of an emergency is a determinant in minimizing mortality rates. It is during flight and the time immediately after arrival in camps or other relief stations that the highest mortality takes place (Sphere Project, 2000). It is also during the first stage of emergencies when people who are on the move or under the trauma of arrival in camps do not have appropriate food preparation utensils and facilities, and hence must rely on ready-to-eat EFPs. This has been the rationale behind the development of various compact EFPs currently produced in other countries (Grobler-Tanner, 2001; Young et al., 1988).

## Target Populations for an Emergency Relief Food Product

Although food relief situations involve people of all ages, there are differences in the composition of populations affected by various types of emergencies. Natural and man-made disasters, on one hand, affect the entire population in the disaster area. Complex emergencies, on the other hand, may affect groups within a population in ways that differ depending on gender, age, or ethnic group. Situations that involve combat, for example, may result in displacement of women and children while older boys and adult men stay behind. UNHCR provisional statistics indicate that there were slightly more women than men among refugee and IDP populations in 2000 (52 vs. 48 percent, respectively). Infants aged 0 to 4 and youngsters aged 5 to 17 years constituted more than 14 and 31 percent, respectively, of the total refugee population, whereas the proportion corresponding to the elderly (aged 60 and above) constituted 8 percent. The largest group was, by far, adults aged 18 to 59, who comprised 46 percent of refugees (UNHCR, 2001).

Population composition in terms of age, sex, health, nutritional status, activity level, and climate are important considerations to ensure that food relief properly addresses the nutritional needs of intended recipients. However, clear international guidelines currently available for estimating food rations for refugees refer mostly to foods provided through the stable supply pipeline that relief agencies establish after the initial stages of an emergency. Little has been published on the appropriate composition of a high-energy, nutrient-dense EFP for use at the onset of emergencies before the food supply system has been established.

The energy level of emergency food rations, in contrast, has been defined. A 1995 report by IOM, also sponsored by USAID, estimated the mean per capita energy requirements (EMPCER) for planning emergency food aid rations at 2,100 kcal (IOM, 1995). This level refers to the average daily energy requirement of individuals in a "typical" population in developing areas of the world, engaged in a light level of physical activity. The estimated EMPCER in the report was based on the following assumptions:

> (1) the population is distributed as indicated in the World Population Profile 1994 report for developing countries; (2) the average height of adult males of 170 cm and of adult females of 155 cm, which are the approximate heights of average males and females in sub-Saharan Africa and slightly greater that those of adults in South and Southeast Asia; (3) the weights of these adults are at the median for U.S. adults of the stated heights; and (4) the total energy expenditure of the adults is 1.55 and 1.56 times the BMR [basal metabolic rate] for males and females, respectively, which is consistent with a light level of activity. (p. 24)

The report did not elaborate on potential food sources to provide that level of energy or on formulations for such rations.

Given that the EFP under study is for use during the initial stages of all types of emergencies when there would be few or no other sources of food or when the prevailing conditions would not be amenable to preparation of other foods, the EFP composition must satisfy the nutritional needs of the subgroup in the population with the greatest needs. In so doing, it can then be assumed that the needs of other population groups—with the notable exception of nursing infants up to 6 month of age, for whom human milk is best—would also be covered by the EFP. USAID requested that the EFP specified by the subcommittee not be a therapeutic food product, although, as mentioned earlier, its eventual use as a supplemental source of nutrients in other feeding programs is possible.

## U.S. Food Relief Programs and Emergency Relief Operations

The United States is the largest donor of humanitarian assistance. The U.S. government contributes to emergency relief and humanitarian assistance in response to natural disasters, man-made disasters, and complex humanitarian emergencies mainly through USAID. This agency's 2000 Performance Report (USAID, 2000a) lists promoting humanitarian assistance as its goal number 6 and states that in 1999, "... the Bureau for Humanitarian Response's Office of U.S. Foreign Disaster Assistance (OFDA) responded to 65 declared disasters in more than 63 countries. These included 17 complex humanitarian emergencies, 41 natural disasters, and 7 man-made disasters." As a result, $294 million was allocated in 1999 to these efforts compared to $186 million in 1998. In addition, the Office of Food for Peace provided $513 million in food assistance for these declared disasters (USAID, 2000b)

Other U.S. agencies coordinate disaster response with USAID, including the Centers for Disease Control and Prevention of the U.S. Department of Health and Human Services, the U.S. Geological Survey of the U.S. Department of the Interior, the National Oceanic and Atmospheric Administration of the U.S. Department of Commerce, and DOD. DOD often provides logistic and personnel support to U.S. relief operations, particularly when rapid airlift of emergency food and medical supplies is necessary.

USAID's Office of Food for Peace takes a leading role in defining the modality and extent of the U.S. food aid response. Food aid is procured from U.S. suppliers and shipped from the United States to the emergency sites. If there is an ongoing food relief program sponsored by USAID in a country neighboring the emergency, available food may be rapidly transferred to the emergency area.

From the operational standpoint, USAID normally provides emergency food assistance directly through U.S. private voluntary organizations (PVOs) and local nongovernmental organizations (NGOs), or indirectly through the World Food Program (WFP). USAID or WFP handles the logistics and the PVOs or NGOs identify the recipients and their needs. However, rapid response in the aftermath of catastrophic events is often undertaken with the cooperation of DOD.

The United States provides emergency food assistance through two programs, Title II of the Food for Peace Program under P.L. 480, which is administered by USAID, and under a surplus disposal program administered by the U.S. Department of Agriculture (USDA), section 416(b) of the Agricultural

Development Act of 1949. All food used in the food assistance programs, including 36 commodities (USAID, 2001b) as well as all other food products—including such foods as the EFP under study—are procured solely by USDA's Commodity Credit Corporation through public solicitation of bids from food producers, distributors, or manufacturers.

The importance of having specifications for a high-energy, nutrient-dense EFP for manufacture in the United States lies in the severe regulatory restrictions that USAID faces for purchasing non-U.S. products. Because there are no American suppliers of EFPs for the agency to purchase under P.L. 480, such products must be purchased abroad using very limited funds available to the agency for non-U.S. purchases. Purchases are made as the need arises, thus incurring long delays in the delivery of desperately needed food relief during emergencies. These factors not only severely limit the amounts that can be purchased, but in the past have forced USAID to forego stockpiling and prepositioning of EFPs at strategic locations around the world for rapid delivery. In contrast, funds from Title II could be used to purchase up to several hundred metric tons of EFPs needed per year if EFPs from U.S. manufacturers were available, and they could be prepositioned to optimize emergency response. Thus, the availability of a U.S.-manufactured EFP that is easily delivered and consumed without further preparation, and appropriately formulated to fulfill the nutritional requirements of individuals undergoing severe physical and mental stress, would undoubtedly facilitate a wider and more rapid response to emergencies by U.S. relief agencies. It could also mean the difference between life and death to thousands of individuals. Developing specifications for such a product is consistent with the passionate appeal for appropriate food for refugees made by Mason and colleagues (1992) and it is also, by any humanitarian measure, a worthy endeavor.

## REFERENCES

Burkholder B, Spiegel P, Salama P. 2001. Methods of determining mortality in the mass displacement and return of emergency-affected populations in Kosovo, 1998–1999. In: Reed HE, Keely CB, eds. *Forced Migration and Mortality*. Washington, DC: National Academy Press. Pp. 86–101.

Crisp J. 2000. Africa's refugees: Patterns, problems and policy changes. Working Paper No. 28. New Issues in Refugee Research. Geneva: United Nations High Commissioner for Refugees.

de Onis M. 2000. Measuring nutritional status in relation to mortality. *Bull World Health Organ* 78:1271–1274.

Grobler-Tanner C. 2001. *A Study of Emergency Relief Foods for Refugees and Displaced Persons*. Washington, DC: U.S. Agency for International Development.

IOM (Institute of Medicine). 1995. *Estimated Mean per Capita Energy Requirements for Planning Emergency Food Aid Rations*. Washington, DC: National Academy Press.

Keely CB, Reed HE, Waldman RJ. 2001. Understanding mortality patterns in complex humanitarian emergencies. In: Reed HE, Keely CB, eds. *Forced Migration and Mortality*. Washington, DC: National Academy Press. Pp. 1–37.

Mason J, Gillespie S, Clugston G, Greaves P. 1992. Misconception on nutrition of refugees. *Lancet* 340:1354.

Snow RW, Craig M, Deichmann U, Marsh K. 1999. Estimating mortality, morbidity and disability due to malaria among Africa's non-pregnant population. *Bull World Health Organ* 77: 624–640.

Sphere Project. 2000. *The Sphere Humanitarian Charter and Minimum Standards in Disaster Response*. Oxford, UK: OXFAM.

UNEP (United Nations Environmental Program). 1992. *Agenda 21*. Online. Available at www.unep.org/Documents/Default.asp?DocumentID=52. Accessed June 13, 2001.

UNHCR (United Nations High Commissioner for Refugees). 2001. *Provisional Statistics on Refugees and Others of Concern to UNHCR for the Year 2000*. Online. Available at www.unhcr.org. Accessed June 20, 2001.

USAID (U.S. Agency for International Development). 2000a. *USAID 2000 Performance Report*. Washington, DC: USAID.

USAID. 2000b. *U.S. International Food Assistance Report 1999*. Washington, DC: USAID.

USAID. 2001a. *Commodities Reference Guide*. Online. Available at www.usaid.gov/hum_response/crg/sec1.htm. Accessed June 15, 2001.

USAID. 2001b. *USAID Humanitarian Response*. Online. Available at www.usaid.gov/hum_response/. Accessed June 12, 2001.

USCR (United States Committee for Refugees). 2000. *Worldwide Refugee Information*. Online. Available at http://www.refugees.org/world/statistics/wrs00_table_asylum2.htm. Accessed June 12, 2001.

Young H, Owen M, Clark J. 1988. A comparison of biscuits used in emergency relief feeding programmes in Ethiopia and Eastern-Sudan 1985/86. *Eur J Clin Nutr* 42:261–271.

# 2

# Nutrient Content and Special Considerations

This chapter presents the rationale for the levels of individual nutrients recommended for the emergency food product (EFP) described in this report, and discusses additional issues to be considered.

> The goal of an EFP is to reduce morbidity and mortality among displaced persons by providing a nutritionally complete food that will be adequate as a sole source of nutrients for as long as 15 days from the recognized time of displacement. It should provide nutrition for the period between initial displacement and establishment of a more stable food supply line.

The EFP should be consumed with an ample quantity of water to ensure that the osmotic load provided by the EFP is diluted. This report assumes that emergency relief agencies will provide potable water supplies as a top priority. This assumption is based on assurances provided by the United States Agency for International Development.

There are five characteristics critical to the development of a successful EFP, listed in order of priority: (1) safe, (2) palatable, (3) easy to deliver, (4) easy to use, and (5) nutritionally complete. This order of priority should guide decisions about competing characteristics in developing a prototype EFP.

**TABLE 2-1** The Population Distribution from Two Reports Providing Demographic Information used to Determine Nutritional Needs for Disaster Responses

| Sub-Saharan Africa[a] | | The Sphere Project[b] | |
|---|---|---|---|
| Age Group (yr) | % of Population | Age Group (yr) | % of Population |
| 0–3 | 10 | 0–4 | 12 |
| 4–6 | 7 | 5–9 | 11 |
| 7–9 | 7 | 10–14 | 11 |
| 10–17 | 17 | 15–19 | 9 |
| 18–60 | 48 | 20–59 | 49 |
| > 60 | 7 | 60+ | 7 |
| | | Pregnant | 2 |
| | | Lactating | 3 |
| | | Male/female | 51/49 |

[a] Jamison and Hobbs (1994).
[b] Sphere Project (2001).

## INTRODUCTION

The nutritional advantages of a single EFP as opposed to two or more products are evident. Providing a limited selection of commodity-type foods may increase the risk of malnutrition because nutritional components that are found in only one of the foods (e.g., ascorbic acid) may be absent from the diet if that food is not selected. Under emergency conditions, diets are invariably highly monotonous, and often relief foods quickly become a medium of exchange and are commonly sold or traded for other foods, water, firewood, alcohol, and a variety of other goods and services. If a nutritionally complete food ration is divided among two or more different foods, or if foods are targeted to specific individuals such as children or pregnant women, then certain foods are more likely to be exchanged. This type of exchange can deprive the population of a portion of the profile of nutrients provided by the emergency food ration and increase the risk of malnutrition. Providing a single ration product would reduce this risk.

## CHARACTERISTICS OF TARGET POPULATIONS

Characteristics of potential target populations were considered in determining the nutrient composition of the EFP. As shown in Table 2-1, some target populations may have as much as 23 percent of the population below 10 years of age and 12 to 17 percent below 5 years of age (Jamison and Hobbs, 1994; Sphere Project, 2001). Refugee groups fleeing from military conflicts may have

**TABLE 2-2** Estimated Mean Per Capita Energy Requirement (EMPCER) by Body Size of Adults

| | Sub-Saharan Africa | South and Southeast Asia | United States |
|---|---|---|---|
| Male height, weight | 170 cm, 63.5 kg | 165 cm, 60.1 kg | 180.4 cm, 78.1 kg |
| Female height, weight | 155 cm, 50.0 kg | 153 cm, 49.0 kg | 163.7 cm, 55.3 kg |
| EMPCER | 2,076 | 2,045 | 2,194 |

SOURCE: Institute of Medicine (IOM, 1995b).

women and children as a large proportion of the population, with only a small proportion of women pregnant or lactating.

Data from the Nutrition Collaborative Research Support Program (CRSP) in Kenya (Calloway et al., 1992; Neumann and Harrison, 1994; Neumann et al., 1991), as well as data from sub-Saharan Africa (Sphere Project, 2001) and South and Southeast Asia (James and Schofield, 1990), indicate that people from these areas have smaller body sizes than those in Western populations (Table 2-2).

While the EFP might have nonemergency uses (e.g., as a complementary food for breast-fed children 7 to 12 months of age), it has been designed as a sole food source for periods of 2 to 15 days. It is likely that the recipient population will be in poor nutritional status and may have some wasting, appetite depression, and malabsorption. The goal of this report is to provide recommendations for a product that would meet the needs of diverse populations.

### General Assumptions

Given the goal outlined above, the following assumptions are made regarding the recipient population:

- The relief food product is the only food consumed.
- Individuals eat to meet their energy requirement.
- Individuals in the target population are of smaller stature and body mass than similarly aged groups in the North American population (this is the same premise used in an earlier report from the Food and Nutrition Board, *Estimated Mean per Capita Energy Requirements for Planning Emergency Food Aid Rations* [IOM, 1995b]).
- All individuals over the age of 6 months will consume the product.

## Estimating Energy Requirements

The energy content of the EFP should be determined by the energy needs of the recipient population. However, because the EFP must be manufactured prior to knowing where it will be needed, the population's energy needs will not be known. Recommended intakes for nutrients from recent reports in the United States and Canada are typically used as the standard for nutrient requirements and thus nutrient content (IOM, 1997a, 1998, 2000, 2001), but, as discussed earlier, energy consumption per individual may be less in the EFP target population than in the United States or Canada due to lower body weights for similar subgroups. Furthermore, because the EFP is a single food meant to support a heterogeneous population, nutrient content must be determined on an energy density basis.

### Estimating Energy Requirements of the Population

A potential basis for calculating the energy requirements for a refugee population is provided in the Institute of Medicine report, *Estimated Mean per Capita Energy Requirements for Planning Emergency Food Aid Rations* (IOM, 1995b). The goal of this report was to establish an estimated mean per capita energy requirement (EMPCER) when little was known about the characteristics of the population. Energy requirements for 14 age and gender groups, plus pregnant and lactating women, were estimated based on body mass and assumptions about energy needs in pregnancy and lactation obtained in two refugee populations. The estimated energy requirements for adults were calculated based on an estimate of basal metabolic rate (BMR) and a physical activity level (PAL). To estimate BMR, the report used equations developed by the Food and Agriculture Organization/World Health Organization/United Nations University (FAO/WHO/UNU, 1985). An average height of 170 cm for adult men and 155 cm for adult women was assumed (the average of adult men and women in sub-Saharan Africa; see Table 2-2). These average heights are slightly greater than those of adults in South and Southeast Asia (Table 2-2) and less than those of the U.S. population. The weights used for the estimates of BMR were the median weight for U.S. adult males of 170 cm (63.5 kg) and females of 155 cm (50 kg). The U.S. median weights (NRC, 1989) were used to provide a conservative estimate of the EMPCER for populations in most developing countries (IOM, 1995b).

For individuals under 18 years of age, values were based on data from affluent populations. Although the individuals from whom these data were derived were larger (and therefore assumed to have a greater BMR) than many children and adolescents from refugee populations, this "extra" allotment for children in developing countries was deemed appropriate on the basis that the additional food would allow some compensatory growth (IOM, 1995b). Both the adult and child values were recognized as overestimates of energy requirements, but were justified in order to establish a conservative EMPCER.

The resulting EMPCER in the report was 2,100 kcal/day (after rounding). This number is used below as the basis for the total energy content of the EFP.

## Estimating Energy Requirements for Specific Life Stage and Gender Groups

The IOM (1995b) report estimated energy requirements for specific life stage and gender groups, as described above. However, it was determined that using that approach was inappropriate for determining the content of the EFP for three reasons. First, the approach could lead to underestimates of nutrient density needed because the nutrient density is based on an assumed energy intake. If energy intake is less than expected, the nutrient density will be too low to meet the micronutrient requirements. Second, the life stage and gender groups do not correspond to the current groups used in the Dietary Reference Intake (DRI) reports (IOM, 1997a, 1998, 2000, 2001). Third, the FAO/WHO/UNU (1985) equations used for infants and children under age 5 are now recognized as flawed (Butte, 1996; Torun et al., 1996).

For the above reasons, estimates of energy requirements for each life stage category were recalculated and are shown in Table 2-3. For individuals 4 years of age and older, estimated energy requirements were obtained by first calculating individual BMRs based on the age, sex, weight, and physiological status of each individual (FAO/WHO/UNU, 1985). Individual energy requirements were then calculated using the same PAL values (women: 1.56, men: 1.55) that were used by IOM (1995b).

With the exception of infants aged 7 through 12 months, the BMR and energy requirements were derived using anthropometric data from individuals in the Kenya Nutrition CRSP (Calloway et al., 1992; Neumann and Harrison, 1994; Neumann et al., 1991). Because the Kenya Nutrition CRSP did not collect anthropometry on children aged 6 through 12 months, the value for this age group was the mean weight of rural infants aged 9 months from the Mexico Nutrition CRSP (Allen et al., 1992).

The Kenya data set contains anthropometry on 1,717 individuals aged 0 to 65 years. As is common in much of the developing world, most adults and children in this population were smaller than U.S. individuals, the result of early growth stunting (Martorell and Habicht, 1986) (Figure 2-1). Additionally, the rural Kenyan population was subject to periodic food shortages and were relatively thin (Neumann and Harrison, 1994).

*Estimating Energy Requirements for Infants and Children.* Recent research using doubly labeled water to measure energy expenditure suggests that values derived from the FAO/WHO/UNU 1985 equations are inflated for infants and young children (Butte, 1996; Butte et al., 2000; de Bruin et al., 1998; Prentice et al., 1988). Therefore, the energy requirements for infants 9 months of age (representing the 7- through 12-month-old group) and children 2 years of age

**TABLE 2-3** Median Weights, Estimated Basal Metabolic Rate (BMR), and Energy Requirements of a Rural Kenyan Population[a]

| Age | Gender | Weight (kg) | BMR (kcal/d) | Energy (kcal/d) | Estimated Number of Emergency Food Product (EFP) Bars[b] per day |
|---|---|---|---|---|---|
| 7–12 mo[c,d] | Both | 7.0 | 371 | 578 | 1–2[e] |
| 1–3 yr[d] | Both | 10.2 | 571 | 855 | 3–4 |
| 4–8 yr | Both | 19.4 | 936 | 1,456 | 6–7 |
| 9–13 yr | Both | 26.5 | 1,086 | 1,693 | 7–8 |
| 14–18 yr | Boys | 42.0 | 1,378 | 2,136 | 9 |
| | Girls | 40.9 | 1,238 | 1,931 | 8–9 |
| 19–50 yr | Men | 54.3 | 1,509 | 2,339 | 9–10 |
| | Women | 51.0 | 1,264 | 1,972 | 8–9 |
| 51+ yr | Men | 56.1 | 1,451 | 2,249 | 9–10 |
| | Women | 47.0 | 1,237 | 1,929 | 8–9 |

[a] Weights from Kenya Nutrition CRSP (Calloway et al., 1992).

[b] Each EFP bar has approximately 233 kcal; 9 bars = 2,100 kcal = one average ration per day. Each can be broken in half to yield 116 kcal. This allows distribution to young children.

[c] Weights from Mexico Nutrition CRSP (Allen et al., 1992).

[d] BMR estimate based on equations of Butte and coworkers (2000).

[e] It is assumed that the EFP would be used as a complementary energy source to human milk and therefore would provide 50 percent of the estimated energy need.

(representing the 1- through 3-year-old group) were calculated according to the formula of Butte and coworkers (2000):

**Energy requirements (MJ/d) = 0.321 + 0.013 × age (mo) - 0.047 × sex + 0.139 × feeding group + 0.277 × weight,**

where sex is coded as 1 for boys, and 2 for girls, and feeding group is coded as 1 for breast-feeding (nearly all children in the Kenyan and Mexican populations). Values for boys and girls were later averaged.

The Butte equations were based on breast-fed children in the United States and yielded values of similar magnitude to those derived for Mexican infants and young children: 638 kcal/day for 0- through 9-month-old infants and 843 kcal/day for 1- through 2-year-old toddlers (Butte et al., 2000). The resulting energy estimates are lower than those used in the IOM (1995b) report (800 and 1,350 kcal/day, respectively), because the IOM values are based on the energy requirements of children derived from the FAO/WHO/UNU (1985) equations and U.S. body weights.

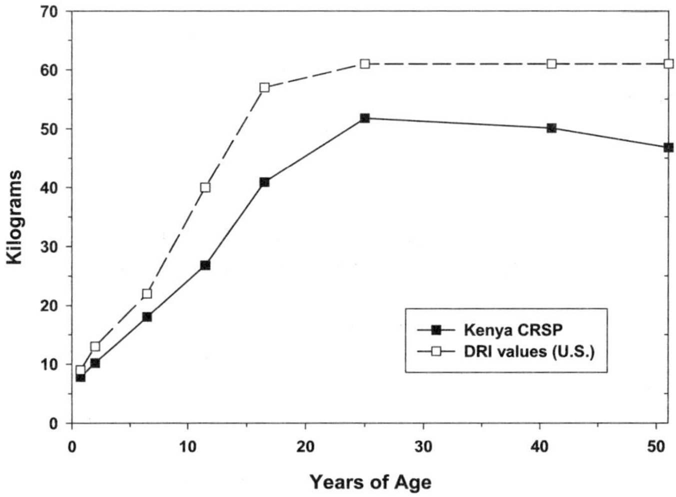


**FIGURE 2-1** Reference weights of DRI life stage groups (U.S. population), and weights of rural Kenyans.

*Estimating Energy Requirements for Pregnancy and Lactation.* Although adequate nutrition during pregnancy and lactation are of concern in refugee populations, the EFP is designed to meet energy requirements based on the assumption that pregnant or lactating women as well as others with higher energy needs (i.e., due to physical activity or rapid growth) will consume additional food bars to meet these needs.

In 1985, FAO/WHO/UNU recommended an increased energy intake of 285 kcal/day during pregnancy. However, the actual increased energy needs during pregnancy vary widely by trimester (Prentice et al., 1996) and by population (Prentice and Goldberg, 2000). For example, the total additional energy needed during pregnancy in The Gambia has been estimated at about 7,000 kcal, or about 25 kcal/day (Prentice and Goldberg, 2000). Moreover, Prentice and colleagues (1996) have proposed that maternal energy metabolism during pregnancy may be lower as measured by change in BMR in women in developing countries versus those in affluent populations. This is believed to be due to their smaller body size. If true, then pregnant women in some emergency feeding situations may not need to consume 285 kcal beyond their nonpregnant, nonlactating energy requirement (or 1 to 2 additional food bars over the 9-bar ration). This number is near to the estimated daily increment of 229 kcal/day during the second trimester, when pregnancy energy requirements appear to be intermediate (Prentice et al., 1996).

FAO/WHO/UNU (1985) also recommended an additional 500 kcal/day during lactation, which assumed an additional 200 kcal/day obtained from maternal fat stores. Prentice and colleagues (1996), based on an extensive review of the literature, recommended an increment of 480 kcal/day for mothers of infants 1 through 6 months of age with previous weight loss.

## CHARACTERISTICS OF THE EMERGENCY RELIEF FOOD PRODUCT

Given the estimated energy requirements (Table 2-3), the proposed energy density for the EFP is 4 to 5 kcal (17 to 21 kJ)/g. To obtain this energy density, an EFP low in water (see Chapter 3) with 35 to 45 percent fat along with 10 to 15 percent protein is required (see sections below). Palatability of the EFP is a primary concern, and should dictate the final choice of ingredients (see Chapter 3). It is assumed that pregnant and lactating women will consume more than the average requirement of 2,100 kcal as needed to support pregnancy and lactation.

### Nutrient Content

The methodology for determining the appropriate amount of each nutrient to be included in the EFP is summarized in Box 2-1, followed by a more detailed explanation and rationale for the approach adopted for each nutrient.

A starting premise for determining the appropriate nutrient content of the EFP is that the upper limit of an individual's food intake is somewhat constrained by his or her total energy requirement, while the lower limit is set by many factors, including appetite, access to food, trading of food, and an individual's ability to make his or her own food decisions. When food intake is lower than energy requirements, the nutrient density may need to be adjusted, thus highlighting a need for testing prototype EFPs developed from the specifications presented in this report.

The recommended intakes (either recommended dietary allowance [RDA] or adequate intake [AI]) as specified in the recent reports on DRIs (IOM, 1997a, 1998, 2000, 2001) were used. These reports provide recommended intakes for vitamins and minerals for 16 life stage and gender groups, plus pregnancy and lactation. It should be noted that these DRIs were established based on a selected criterion or criteria of adequacy consistent with good health, as opposed to the mere prevention of overt deficiencies. Thus the values obtained may be higher than those previously recommended by WHO. RDAs were calculated from the estimates of average requirements (EAR) using an estimate of the variability among individuals in the requirement. In most cases, the coefficient of variation of nutrient requirements was assumed to be 10 percent. The RDA is set at two

**BOX 2-1** Summary of Methodology to Determine the Nutrient Content of the EFP

1. Use the Adequate Intakes (AI), Recommended Dietary Allowances (RDA), and Tolerable Upper Intake Levels (UL) as developed by IOM (1997a, 1998, 2000, 2001) or, for protein, FAO/WHO (2000).
2. Use 2,100 kcal/person as the target for the population, but evaluate the amounts needed based on estimated energy expenditure for different subgroups of the population.
3. Select the life stage and gender group that has the highest nutrient needs relative to estimated energy needs for each nutrient. This group is designated the limiting subgroup.
4. Determine the nutrient density for the limiting subgroup utilizing the AI or RDA by dividing the recommended intake of the nutrient by the energy requirement determined for that subgroup (see Table 2-3).
5. Adjust the nutrient density value of the limiting subgroup based on probable malabsorption, bioavailability assumptions, potential nutrient interactions, and properties related to the plant sources of ingredients utilized in the EFP.
6. Determine for each nutrient if the requirement for the limiting subgroup exceeds the UL for any other age group.
7. Adjust the proposed nutrient level, if necessary, to ensure that the UL is not reached for other age groups. If the rationale used allows some subgroups to exceed the UL, so state. Provide a maximum level for the EFP based on the UL.
8. Recommend food ingredients that would prevent interactions with other nutrients and avoid reaching the maximum value.
9. Describe the assumptions and the scientific rationale underlying the recommended level for each nutrient.

standard deviations above the EAR, and should meet the requirements of almost all of the U.S. and Canadian populations for which it is recommended.

For some required nutrients, it was not possible to establish an intake at which half of a life stage and gender group would be adequately nourished, while the other half would demonstrate signs of inadequacy. Thus an EAR could not be set. However, data were available that could be used to establish a level of intake that appeared adequate for most, if not all, people consuming that amount. This is called the *adequate intake* (AI). AIs are available for a number of the nutrients included in the EFP. Given that the data upon which an AI is based are less certain, there is more judgment in its derivation. In some cases, the EFP may not provide the AI level due to constraints related to palatability or cost. In this case, the probability that the target population has underlying nutrient deficiencies is assumed, and what is feasible for a product to be used for 10 to 15 days as the sole source of nutrition is determined.

There are also nutrients that are deemed essential for inclusion in an EFP, but for which DRIs have not yet been determined. In this case (i.e., macronutrients and electrolytes), other recommendations for these nutrients (FAO/WHO, 2000; NRC, 1989) were considered in determining the amounts appropriate for the EFP.

Ideally, the formulation of an EFP requires information on variability in actual consumption of the relief food. Since such information is not available at this developmental stage of the product, a few cautionary flags must be raised in the use of the proposed EFP:

- The EFP is not designed to meet all the nutrient needs for pregnancy and lactation; however, due to the energy requirements being conservatively estimated based on energy needs for smaller individuals, it should meet the requirements for most nutrients for almost all women.
- The EFP is not appropriate for severely malnourished individuals who require medical attention. Severe malnutrition is defined in the WHO Sick Child Initiative as quoted by IOM (1995a) as the presence of any one of the following symptoms: visible severe wasting, severe pallor, clouding of the cornea, or edema of both feet.
- The EFP is not a therapeutic nutritional supplement. (A ration distributed to the general population cannot be formulated as a therapeutic diet, as it would present too many risks of excess intake for individuals who were not severely malnourished. Severely malnourished individuals need special help, including fluid and electrolyte replacement therapy, blood transfusions for severe anemia, and medical supervision. This food product is *not* meant to be a substitute for this therapy, but a sustaining ration for people who have been uprooted due to war or natural disaster.)
- The EFP is not a substitute for human milk for infants agers 0 to 6 months.
- The EFP is not designed to meet the needs of young infants; however, it may be combined with water to produce a gruel suitable as a complementary food for older infants (7 to 12 months of age).

### Determination of a Minimal Nutrient Density

At the population level, there are a number of individual minimal nutrient densities for each nutrient. If a single food must meet the nutrient requirement of most individuals in the population, this food should have a nutrient density that meets or exceeds the minimal nutrient densities of most individuals in the population. Since food intake is limited by energy requirements, a high nutrient density is necessary to meet the nutrient requirements of an individual with low energy needs. The approach described here to establish the nutrient content for the EFP provides a complete food for individuals consuming on average as little as 855 kcal/day (1- to 3-year-old age group) to those who may require in excess of the average ration of 2,100 kcal/day (adult men); thus the EFP can be used by a diverse population.

The approach used to determine nutrient density for the EFP is as follows: for each nutrient, a minimal density value was estimated for the life stage and gender group in the population with the highest nutrient requirement relative to their energy requirement using the data on recommended nutrient intakes (Table 2-4) (IOM, 1997a, 1998, 2000, 2001; NRC, 1989; WHO, 2000), divided by the estimated average energy requirement for that life stage and gender group based on data from Kenyan refugee populations (Table 2-3). Neither pregnant nor lactating women were considered as a limiting group because for some nutrients (e.g., iodine, vitamin A) the minimal nutrient density would provide intakes that would exceed the UL (IOM, 1997a) for other groups in the population. Additional assumptions used in setting the minimal nutrient density include:

- The relief food is the only food consumed.
- Individual energy consumption equals energy requirement.
- The food product should provide a nutrient density that will meet the nutrient requirements of almost all members of each life stage and gender group without exceeding the UL for any group.

These assumptions err in the direction of providing more of a nutrient than may be necessary unless energy consumption does not meet energy requirements. In most cases, the RDA values used were calculated from EARs which were originally estimated from only a few individuals with assumed variations in requirements, and then extrapolated to other age and gender groups using conservative approaches. Most of the estimates of AIs were based on mean intakes for healthy population groups that did not demonstrate any indicators of inadequacy of the nutrient, and thus could easily be overestimates of actual requirements for subgroups.

Finally, in the case of many nutrients, the minimal nutrient density was subsequently modified upward in order to ensure that possible interactions with other nutrients or storage conditions, poorer bioavailability, or assumed presence of diarrhea or disease in the recipient population were taken into account. Since increased amounts of nutrients will increase the cost and potentially may affect palatability and shelf life of the EFP, and palatability is the major factor that ensures adequate energy consumption, slight reductions in these recommended amounts may be necessary.

**TABLE 2-4** Unadjusted Baseline Minimal Nutrient Density Values Using Recommended Intakes

| Nutrient | Limiting Group | Baseline per 1,000 kcal[a] | Basis for Recommended Intake |
|---|---|---|---|
| Fat | N/A | 39–50 g | Providing an energy density of 4–5 kcal/g |
| Protein[b] | 51+ yr, men | 34 g | Balance studies |
| Carbohydrate | N/A | 100–125 g | Seven to 12 of the 23–35 g of total carbohydrate should be from sugars for adequate palatability |
| Sodium[c] | 2–5 yr, children | 1.3 g | Maximum level of intake |
| Potassium[c] | 2–5 yr, children | 1.7 g | Level estimated to meet minimum requirements |
| Chloride[c] | 2–5 yr, children | 2.0 g | Level estimated to be equimolar to sodium |
| Calcium | 9–13 yr, children | 768 mg | Based on maximal calcium retention |
| Phosphorus | 9–13 yr, children | 740 mg | Based on factorial approach |
| Magnesium | 14–18 yr, boys | 190 mg | Amount needed to maintain magnesium balance |
| Chromium | — | 13.5 μg | Based on amounts in well-balanced diets/1,000 kcal |
| Copper | 51+ yr, women | 470 μg | Biochemical indicators of copper status |
| Iodine | 1–3 yr, children | 105 μg | Balance studies |
| Iron[d] | 19–50 yr, women | 9 mg | Based on iron requirement (estimated basal losses, increase in hemoglobin mass, increase in nonstorage iron, increase in storage iron) plus assumed iron absorption |
| Manganese | 1–3 yr, children | 1.4 mg | Average intake in healthy population |
| Selenium | 14–18 yr, girls | 28 μg | Maximizing plasma glutathione peroxidase activity |
| Zinc | 14–18 yr, boys | 5.2 mg | Level needed to match exogenous losses |
| Vitamin A | 14–18 yr, boys | 420 μg RAE | Level needed to maintain adequate stores |
| Vitamin D | 51–70 yr, women | 5.2 μg | Maintain serum 25(OH)vitamin D levels |
| Vitamin E | 14–18 yr, girls | 7.8 mg | Level needed to prevent hydrogen peroxide-induced hemolysis |

*continued*

**TABLE 2-4** Continued

| Nutrient | Limiting Group | Baseline per 1,000 kcal[a] | Basis for Recommended Intake |
|---|---|---|---|
| Vitamin K | 19–50 yr, men | ~60 μg | Average intakes in adequately nourished population groups |
| Vitamin C | 51+ yr, men | 40 mg | Level needed to maintain near-maximal neutrophil concentration with minimal urinary loss |
| Thiamin | 1–3 yr, children | 0.6 mg | Level needed for normal erythrocyte transketolase activity |
| Riboflavin | 14–18 yr, boys | 0.6 mg | Level needed to maintain normal erythrocyte glutathione reductase activity and urinary riboflavin excretion |
| Niacin | 14–18 yr, boys | 7.5 mg NE | Level needed to maintain adequate niacin metabolism as measured by excretion of metabolites |
| Vitamin $B_6$ | 51+ yr, women | 0.8 mg | Level needed to replete depleted stores |
| Folate[e] | 14–18 yr, girls | 207 μg | Level needed to maintain normal homocysteine, red cell folate concentrations |
| Vitamin $B_{12}$ | 14–18 yr, girls | 1.2 μg | Level needed to maintain normal $B_{12}$ levels and hematological status in adults |
| Pantothenic acid | 14–18 yr, girls | 2.6 mg | Average intake in healthy population |
| Biotin | 51+, women | 16 μg | Average intake in healthy population |
| Choline | 51+, men | 244 mg | Level needed to maintain normal liver enzyme levels in young adults |

[a] Estimated energy requirements for each limiting group taken from Table 2-3.
[b] From NRC (1989); based on reference weights from IOM (1997a) and estimated energy expenditure from Table 2-3.
[c] Values based on estimated requirements, desirable intakes, or maximal intakes (NRC,1989).
[d] Based on 10% iron bioavailability.
[e] If folate is provided as synthetic folate, which is more readily absorbed, these numbers should be divided by 1.6.
SOURCE: IOM (1997a, 1998, 2000, 2001).

In order to individualize and facilitate the use of the EFP to the extent possible, it is designed to be consumed in multiple subunits so that it is possible to consume from 117 kcal (one-half of a scored 233-kcal EFP bar) to 2,100 kcal (9 EFP bars, which are 1 day's ration) or more (e.g., pregnant or lactating women or individuals with high energy expenditure) over the entire day, yet still contain adequate nutrient levels to meet the needs of smaller individuals with lower energy intakes.

Although there are conflicting data on whether individuals will consume enough of a single, biscuit-type food product to meet their energy requirements (Brown et al., 1995; Sanchez-Griñan et al., 1992), it is assumed for the purpose of this report that individuals, at least for a short period of time, will consume enough EFPs to meet their energy requirements. The nutrient content of the EFP is based on this assumption.

## NUTRIENTS INCLUDED IN THE EMERGENCY RELIEF FOOD PRODUCT SPECIFICATIONS

For each nutrient or nutrient group that follows, the assumptions, including the minimal nutrient density, the limiting groups, and how the RDA, AI, or other values were utilized are discussed. Since the EFP will be used for a wide range of age groups, in those cases where maximum values were set, they were developed from the UL values included in the DRI reports (IOM 1997a, 1998, 2000, 2001).

### Energy-Yielding Nutrients

Fat, protein, and carbohydrates comprise the energy nutrients. The rationale for the fat, protein, and carbohydrate levels in the EFP are discussed below.

#### Dietary Fat

The recommended fat content of the EFP is 35 to 45 percent of calories and takes into consideration the following:

- the quantity of fat needed to provide a food of sufficient energy density to meet energy requirements, to be lightweight, and to be palatable;
- the quantity of fat needed to ensure adequate absorption of fat-soluble vitamins;
- the quality of fat needed to provide an adequate supply of essential fatty acids; and
- the ability to protect fat from oxidation and degradation under severe storage and transport conditions.

The maximum fat content of the EFP is limited by the minimal requirements for other macronutrients, vitamins, and minerals (Jéquier, 1999; Koletzko, 1999). The principal mechanisms for increasing the energy density of a food are to either reduce water content or to increase fat content. Because fat on a weight basis is 2.25 times as energy dense as either carbohydrate or protein, a high-fat product will weigh less than lower-fat products of similar water and energy content. The reduced weight of an energy-dense food also has advantages with respect to storage and transport. Furthermore, infants and young children have comparatively high energy requirements per kilogram of body weight (Koletzko, 1999) and have limited capacities to consume food. Therefore, very-low-fat diets increase the risk of inadequate energy intakes that would result in inadequate intakes of some micronutrients in young children. FAO/WHO (1994) suggested diets of children under 2 years of age should contain 30 to 40 percent of energy from fat.

*Satiation.* High-fat foods are readily over-consumed, and experimental studies suggest little effect of fat per se on satiation (feeling of fullness) when energy density of the meal is held constant (Rolls, 2000; Rolls and Bell, 1999; Saltzman et al., 1997; Stubbs et al., 1996; van Stratum et al., 1978). These results suggest that an energy-dense food, regardless of fat content, is less likely to induce satiation, and therefore is likely to promote consumption of greater amounts of energy. In the case of a refugee population, in which anorexia may be common, the provision of a higher-fat, nutrient-dense food may be an important means of ensuring adequate energy intake.

*Palatability.* The fat content of a food can have a significant influence on its sensory properties and the quantity of the food that is consumed (Drewnowski, 1997). Fat contributes to flavor, mouth feel, moistness, and other textural properties, depending on the food and the type of fat. Relatively little research has been published concerning the influence of fat content on the palatability of products similar to the proposed EFP. Recently, Abdallah and coworkers (1998) asked 102 men to rate the pleasantness of 39 commercially available cookies and cakes. Sugar content was the best predictor of pleasantness. However, the highest ratings of pleasantness occurred with foods that were high in both sugar and fat. Moisture content bore little relationship to pleasantness after statistically controlling for the fat and sugar content of the products. Others have investigated the sensory effects of reducing the fat content of five cookies. Only a reduction of fat by 50 percent of its original recipe was associated with declines in sensory ratings (Drewnowski et al., 1998). In both studies, subjects were much more sensitive to variability in sugar content than in fat content.

*Fat Intake and Absorption of Fat-Soluble Vitamins.* The absorption of fat-soluble vitamins and provitamins is dependent on fat in the diet. However, the precise quantity of dietary fat needed for efficient absorption of fat-soluble vitamins is poorly understood. A common rule of thumb is that fat energy should not fall below 10 percent of total energy (Jéquier, 1999). Thus, the fat content of the EFP is more than adequate to promote absorption of fat-soluble vitamins.

*Type of Fat.* As the nutritional quality of diets in developing countries improves, the availability and the percentage of energy in the diet contributed by fat increases (Tagle, 1988). The greatest concern in developing the EFP regarding type of fat is to include fats/oils that will provide the greatest stability in terms of storage of the finished product, without the inclusion of fat of animal origin. For long-term health, other aspects of dietary fat, such as the proportion of essential fatty acids or the inclusion of long chain polyunsaturated fatty acids (LC-PUFAs) is of interest as well. However, with the limited time that the EFPs will be used (15 days or less), cost and storage requirements of the finished product limit the advisability of including some of these specific fatty acids.

*Polyunsaturated Fatty Acids.* Polyunsaturated fatty acids are necessary for normal health in adults and normal development in the fetus and infant (Uauy et al., 1999). The essential fatty acids, α-linolenic acid (LNA, *n*-3) and linoleic acid (LA, *n*-6), present in various vegetable oils, are precursors for the other *n*-3 and *n*-6 LC-PUFAs. In animal models, synthesis of docosahexaenoic (DHA) and arachidonic acid (AA) from their essential fatty acid precursors are decreased by experimental protein and energy malnutrition (Lopez-Pedrosa et al., 1998; Marin et al., 1995) and observational studies in infants have documented associations between protein–energy malnutrition (PEM) and signs of *n*-6 fatty acid deficiency (Decsi et al., 1998; Holman et al., 1981; Koletzko et al., 1986; Leichsenring et al., 1995; Marin et al., 1991; Smit et al., 1997).

Studies indicate that children with sickle cell anemia and with zinc and copper deficiencies appear to have impaired ability to utilize LA and LNA (Cunnane, 1981; Enomoto et al., 1998). Research has shown considerable regional variability in the LC-PUFA content of human milk of women in developing countries, presumably due to variability in diets (Chulei et al., 1995; Koletzko et al., 1992; Laryea et al., 1995; Okolo et al., 2000; Rocquelin et al., 1998; Schmeits et al., 1999; VanderJagt et al., 2000; Xiang et al., 1999). Of relevance to some developing country populations is the fact that high LA intakes from specific vegetable oils (e.g., corn oil) may decrease the synthesis of DHA from LNA. The recommendation that a ratio of LA to LNA between 5:1 and 10:1 has been made (FAO/WHO, 1994), and seems reasonable and fairly easy to obtain from vegetable oil sources.

Although an EFP having at least 35 percent of calories from vegetable oil sources will probably not be totally devoid of such fatty acids, the constraints of manufacturing, required storage life, and the impact of oxidized unsaturated fat on flavor dictate against addition of these fatty acids.

*Vitamin E, PUFA, and Oxidation.* Because of their susceptibility to oxidation, very high intakes of PUFA, without a correspondingly high intake of antioxidants, can lead to vitamin E deficiency (Valk and Hornstra, 2000). Fortunately, most commonly consumed vegetable oils are good sources of vitamin E (IOM, 2000) and have relatively high vitamin E:PUFA ratios (Dupont et al., 1990). Recommendations to provide adequate vitamin E intakes in high PUFA diets have been made, and vary from 0.4 (NRC, 1989) to 0.6 mg (FAO/WHO, 1994) of α-tocopherol per gram of PUFA.

*Maximum Fat Content of the EFP.* The upper limit of fat for the EFP is recommended to be 45 percent of energy in order to produce a stable product that would not be unduly affected by oxidation.

Fat intakes in developing countries are often quite low and come from a small number of principal dietary sources. Average fat intakes of school-aged children ranged from 10 percent of energy (in rural Kenya where animal products are consumed in relatively small amounts) to 25 percent of energy in peri-urban Egypt (Beaton, 1995). In Kenya, 40 percent of the fat in the diet was polyunsaturated, much of it from corn oil (Calloway et al., 1992). In The Gambia, children's intake of fat as a percent of energy declined from birth and stabilized at 24 months of age, when the average intake of energy from fat was 15 percent (Prentice and Paul, 2000), with most of the fat coming from groundnuts and cereals. This maximum level of fat exceeds the fat content of diets normally consumed in many developing countries, but should enhance palatability of the EFP.

In summary, recommendations regarding the fat content of the EFP are as follows:

- Total fat should comprise 35 to 45 percent of energy.
- Saturated fat should comprise at least 10 percent of energy.
- Total PUFA should be 7 to 10 percent of energy.
- The ratio of linoleic acid to α-linolenic acid should fall between 5:1 and 10:1 derived from a mixture of vegetable oils.

## Protein and Amino Acid Requirements

Protein is essential for all physiological functions. Although two structural proteins, collagen and elastin, comprise about half of the proteins in the adult body, the protein associated with muscle, visceral organs, and blood is the most dynamic and most affected by poor nutritional status (Crim and Munro, 1994). Adults with good nutritional status and in protein balance turn over about 300 g of protein/day (Stein, 1995); growth during childhood and pregnancy increases this turnover. The body has no readily identifiable reserves of amino acids essential for protein synthesis. Loss of 30 to 40 percent of total body protein invariably results in death from starvation (Cahill, 1970). Rapid losses due to lack

**TABLE 2-5** Recommended Amino Acid Pattern of an Emergency Relief Food Product (EFP)

| Nutrient | Amount[a] (mg/kg body weight [BW]) | Amino Acid (mg/g Protein)[c] |
|---|---|---|
| Protein[b] (g/kg BW) | 1.0 | — |
| Isoleucine | 31 | 28 |
| Leucine | 73 | 66 |
| Lysine | 64 | 58 |
| Methionine + cysteine | 27 | 25 |
| Phenylalanine + tyrosine | 69 | 63 |
| Threonine | 37 | 34 |
| Tryptophan | 12.5 | 11 |
| Valine | 38 | 35 |
| Histidine[c] | 8 | 19 |

[a] The amino acid requirement for children 2 years of age was used (NRC, 1989).
[b] Total protein based on 1 g/kg body weight, using reference body weights from the Dietary Reference Intake reports (IOM, 1997a).

of food in emergency situations can thus result in serious health consequences over relatively short periods of time.

PEM may be present in populations that are likely to be recipients of the EFP (Young and Jaspars, 1995). For instance, an August 1989 survey of the Hartisheik A camp in Ethiopia indicated that 15.5 percent of reported cases of death in children less than 5 years of age were due to PEM and general malnutrition (CDC, 1990). The EFP target populations may have reduced energy intakes and low protein intakes, resulting in negative energy and nitrogen balances (Fjeld et al., 1989), reduced growth and/or lactation volume, and loss of body weight and muscle mass (Golden, 1994; Golden et al., 1977; Rice et al., 2000; Young and Jaspars, 1995). Limited muscle mass has been documented by lower body weights and mid-arm circumferences (Collins, 2000; De Onis et al., 2000; Young and Jaspars, 1995). Decreased skeletal muscle mass decreases functional capabilities (Dudley et al., 1989) and may impact the ability to perform normal life functions, as documented with PEM (Day and DeHeer, 2001; Kalra et al., 2001). Thus the EFP must provide adequate protein of appropriate quality.

Protein requirements include two components: the need for amino acids and for total protein (NRC, 1989). The EFP should meet both of these needs. The essential amino acid requirements for 2-year-old children identified by WHO (FAO/WHO/UNU, 1985), and subsequently adopted by the National Research Council (NRC, 1989), serve as the minimum amino acid pattern to use for the

| Amount/233 kcal Food Bar (g) | Amount/1,000 kcal of EFP (g) | Amount/2,100 kcal Ration (g) |
|---|---|---|
| 8 | 34 | 71 |
| 0.22 | 0.95 | 1.99 |
| 0.52 | 2.23 | 4.69 |
| 0.46 | 1.96 | 4.12 |
| 0.20 | 0.84 | 1.78 |
| 0.50 | 2.13 | 4.47 |
| 0.27 | 1.15 | 2.41 |
| 0.09 | 0.37 | 0.78 |
| 0.28 | 1.18 | 2.48 |
| 0.15 | 0.64 | 1.35 |

[c] Amino acid patterns for children 2 to 5 years of age from FAO/WHO/UNU (1985).

EFP (34 g/1,000 kcal, or 8 g/EFP bar) along with the generally recommended amount of total protein of 1 g/kg body weight (see Table 2-5). Although the protein content may be slightly low for young children (their RDA is 1.2 g/kg body weight [NRC, 1989]), the recommendation must take into consideration that a higher protein level per kilocalorie may be too high for adults and may not be as palatable (Young et al., 1985). ***A maximum of 15 percent of total calories as protein is recommended to prevent renal load problems and thirst promotion*** (Briend and Golden, 1993). Thus, the amount of protein recommended for the EFP is a compromise. Although the pattern of amino acids will meet the essential amino acid needs of the young child, the total protein may be limiting.

Because the EFP may be the sole food source for as long as 15 days, ***the protein should have a protein digestibility-corrected amino acid score (PDCAAS) of 1.0 or better*** (FAO/WHO, 1989). The protein and amino acids could be provided by a combination of soybean protein isolates or concentrates and grains such as wheat, and complemented with milk solids (NRC, 1989). If milk solids are used, some amount of lactose would be included, but the level should be kept below 17 g/1,000 kcal (see "Lactose," below).

There is abundant research demonstrating the effectiveness of combinations of plant proteins such as those from soybeans and wheat flour in meeting essential amino acid needs along with total protein (Brown et al., 1982; Clegg, 1960; Dahlin and Lorenz, 1993; Friedman and Brandon, 2001; Grange et al., 1994). Wheat flour has good digestibility and provides the physico-chemical properties for a palatable food product but is limiting in lysine content. Soy protein has lysine and is a high-quality protein, but may be limiting in methionine or sulfur amino acids for children (Friedman and Brandon, 2001). Other legume protein sources may not be sufficient. For example, the combination of wheat flour, chickpeas, and milk powder has a PDCAAS of 0.73 (FAO/WHO, 1989), which is low in lysine. Amino acids should be provided in the EFP only as intact protein and not as free amino acids. ***Supplementing with amino acids is not recommended as it will affect taste and increase cost, and can lead to problems of imbalance without adequate premixing.***

Subsequent food processing should not affect protein quality. For instance, heat used in extrusion could reduce the lysine availability of the product (Clegg, 1960; Dahlin and Lorenz, 1993). ***Protein content in the final EFP should be within 10 percent of specifications.***

## Carbohydrates

Carbohydrates include monosaccharides (glucose, fructose, and galactose); disaccharides (maltose, sucrose, and lactose); oligosaccharides (maltodextrins); and polysaccharides—starch (amylose and amylopectin)—and nonstarch (cellulose, xantham, pectins, and carrageenans) (Bemiller and Whistler, 1996). Carbohydrates serve several functions as components of the EFP. They provide energy, sweetness, and desirable physical properties of the product, and are necessary for sodium absorption to maintain electrolyte status. There are also maximum levels beyond which undigested and unabsorbed carbohydrates result in gastrointestinal problems due to gas production by intestinal bacteria. Carbohydrates and fat are the two major energy sources provided by the EFP; ***carbohydrate should be provided primarily as starch associated with the grains and/or legumes used as protein sources and to meet specific requirements for taste, palatability, stability, and metabolic function*** (FAO/WHO, 1998).

*Sweetness and Physical Properties.* Cookie-like products (e.g., slightly sweet biscuits) have proven to be most acceptable for a wide spectrum of cultures during various emergencies where relief food products have been used, although compressed food bars such as the Norwegian BP-5 were also acceptable (Grobler-Tanner, 2001). The only flavor found to be acceptable to widely diverse populations was sweetness (Drewnowski, 1997; Young et al., 1985). Therefore, nutrient composition recommendations for the EFP include sugars such as sucrose or corn syrup to provide sweetness and to improve the texture of the EFP. The specifications for the EFP limit total sugar levels, however, as described in the following subsections. Most of the carbohydrate in the EFP will be in the form of starch.

*Glucose.* A high incidence of diarrhea and malabsorption, commonly due to poor sanitation, is associated with uprooted populations (UN Subcommittee on Nutrition, 2001). Provision of potable water is the highest priority in emergency relief efforts (UNHCR, 2000), with the EFP as the primary source of electrolytes. Therefore, the emergency food product should provide glucose and sodium in quantities that will optimize intestinal absorption when consumed with ample water, yet not be so high as to be malabsorbed (Santosham et al., 1987).

Ability to absorb glucose in the small intestine and transport it with sodium remains intact during acute diarrhea (Hirschhorn, 1980). The EFP should provide 6 g of glucose for each 1 g of sodium to promote gastrointestinal uptake of sodium (Santosham et al., 1987). The sodium recommendation is 1.4 g/1,000 kcal, thus resulting in a requirement for 8.6 g of free glucose/1,000 kcal. However, the total monosaccharide level must be less than 25 percent of carbohydrates, by weight, to prevent osmotic diarrhea and elevation of the osmotic load. Use of maltodextrins to provide 8.6 g of free glucose is recommended due to the cost of free glucose compared to maltodextrins.

*Lactose.* Milk solids may be used in the EFP, but the level of milk sugar—lactose—needs to be considered. Because there may be a high incidence of adult lactase deficiency in the populations receiving the EFP, consumption of excessive lactose might be a concern if it led to abdominal discomfort, flatulence, abdominal bloating, and diarrhea (Scrimshaw and Murray, 1988). Secondary lactase deficiency also has been shown to be associated with acute gastroenteritis, malnutrition, acquired immune deficiency syndrome enteropathy, and diarrhea of infectious origin in both adults and children (Riley and Marsh, 1998; Scrimshaw and Murray, 1988). Such lactase deficiency may be transient or chronic in nature. For these reasons, ***use of lactose as a carbohydrate source is not recommended.*** Because milk solids provide high-quality protein and often are readily available for emergency feeding programs, their use as a protein source in the EFP may be desirable.

Controlled studies have shown that the majority of individuals demonstrated to be lactose maldigestors do not experience symptoms with 1 cup of milk or the equivalent amount of lactose (12 g) or more consumed at one time (Scrimshaw and Murray, 1988; Suarez et al., 1995). Many of these studies are based on results following ingestion of single test meals providing varying amounts of lactose, and tolerance to repeated intake of this amount of lactose on the same day and over a extended period of time is less clear. However, the reported milk consumption of individuals shown to be lactose maldigestors often exceeds 1 cup/day (Scrimshaw and Murray, 1988). In a controlled study by Calloway and Chenoweth (1973), four subjects shown to be lactose maldigestors were fed a diet that included 1,000 g of homogenized low-fat milk providing approximately 50 g of lactose in four divided doses for a period of 12 days. Breath hydrogen concentrations were slightly or moderately elevated in two of the subjects at this level of intake but there were few subjective complaints of discomfort due to the diet.

Although the EFP is not intended to be used in treatment of individuals with severe diarrhea or malnutrition, the use of products containing milk in feeding adults and children with these conditions demonstrates the acceptability of including milk in emergency rations. Collins and colleagues (1998) recently reported successful use of a product containing dried skim milk, vegetable oil, vitamins, and minerals as part of the diet given to adult patients with severe malnutrition in Baidoa, Somalia. Although the milk product was diluted in the first few days of treatment, the amount was gradually increased and provided 137 or 95 g of lactose/day. The latter diet was reported as being better tolerated but the investigators attributed this response to the lower protein content of the diet rather than the reduced amount of lactose.

The use of diets containing milk in treating young children with diarrhea has been studied extensively (Brown, 1991; Brown et al., 1991; Penny and Brown, 1992). A meta-analysis of clinical trials that compared the outcomes of young children treated with either lactose-containing or lactose-free diets (Brown et al., 1994) showed an overall treatment failure rate of approximately 22 percent among children treated with lactose-containing diets compared with a treatment failure rate of 12 percent among those who received lactose-free diets. On the basis of these meta-analyses the author concluded that the majority of children with acute diarrhea can safely receive undiluted, lactose-containing milks, which would contain about 12 g/240 ml, distributed over multiple feeding episodes. However, children with severe diarrhea and dehydration may have increased treatment failure rates if they receive undiluted lactose-containing milk and should be managed under close supervision. This concern, however, is not applicable to use of the EFP since it is not intended as a therapeutic treatment for individuals with severe diarrhea or malnutrition.

Based on evidence suggesting that consumption of 12 g of lactose contained in 1 cup of milk would be tolerated by populations with a high prevalence of lactose maldigestion when consumed as part of a meal, if approximately one-third of the daily ration of EFPs (and thus one-third of the lactose) is consumed during each eating episode, the maximum lactose content should be 17 g/1,000 kcal (4 g/EFP bar). Thus, children ages 1 to 3 years consuming 855 kcal/day (Table 2-3) would receive approximately 14.5 g/day or ~5 g/meal episode. This amount of lactose would allow milk solids to provide about one-third of the specified content of protein (34 g/1,000 kcal) and one-half of the calcium (768 mg/1,000 kcal) for the EFP. ***Lactose should only be present in the EFP due to its presence in milk solids—it should not be added.***

*Fiber*. Generally, fiber is considered essential for human health, and the targeted population should consume fiber-containing foods if possible (NRC, 1989). However, other requirements of the EFP limit the advisability of its providing fiber. First, it is well recognized that individuals living in sub-Saharan Africa and Asia usually consume about 30 g/day of nonstarch polysaccharides, an indication of adequate fiber intake (FAO/WHO, 1998). The EFP will be used for less than 15 days and hence a lack of fiber would not result in a chronic problem or exacerbate a condition. Furthermore, the energy density of the product needs to be high (e.g., 4.2 kcal/g is the energy density of the BP-5 [Young et al., 1988]) to meet the needs of all age groups in the population, and to facilitate ease of transport and distribution. Consequently, although the EFP will contain some fiber because of its grain and legume constituents, the level of fiber should be limited to provide maximal energy density.

*Importance of Carbohydrates for Physical Activity.* Individuals in need of the EFP may often be walking long distances on foot, or may be expending a large amount of energy erecting shelters, finding water, finding fuel, or meeting hygiene needs. These factors emphasize the importance of carbohydrate in the EFP in a number of ways. First, during moderate-intensity labor (e.g., less strenuous than a brisk walk, under 5.6 km/h, or at less than 40 to 50 percent $VO_{2max}$), the primary metabolic fuel is fat with carbohydrate contributing about 25 percent toward total caloric expenditure (Brooks and Trimmer, 1996). However, during the course of several hours of work, muscle and liver glycogen stores can become depleted and the ability to walk or perform physical tasks declines. Adequate dietary carbohydrate intake is necessary to sustain prolonged exercise of more than 1 hour (Ivy et al., 1979) and to allay fatigue.

Second, if an insufficient amount of carbohydrate is consumed on consecutive days by individuals who exercise for prolonged periods, they likely will experience irritability, dizziness, and/or nausea in addition to fatigue (Sherman, 1983). Moreover, carbohydrate stored in muscle and liver tissue as glycogen involves water storage (i.e., 3 g of water/g of carbohydrate). This water is released when glycogen is metabolized and provides a minor, but useful, contribution to meeting fluid needs. Finally, compared to no feeding, carbohydrate intake during exercise increases endurance (Brooks et al., 2000). The EFP is convenient to eat during periods of physical activity, requires no preparation, and does not significantly divert the consumer from essential daily tasks. Individuals can thus benefit from consuming the EFP before and during periods of prolonged activity because it includes 40 to 50 percent of its calories as carbohydrate. This level of carbohydrate allows for an energy-dense ration (35 to 45 percent from fat) and for adequate protein (10 to 15 percent of energy coming from protein).

To summarize carbohydrate requirements for the EFP per 1,000 kcal/day:

- 40 to 50 percent of energy as carbohydrate, at least 50 percent of which is from starch;
- no more than 25 percent of carbohydrates as monosaccharides;
- at least 8.6 g of glucose from maltodextrins to allow for sodium transport;
- no more than 17 g of lactose from milk solids (no free lactose added) per 1,000 kcal;
- primary role for sucrose or corn syrup is to provide palatability and texture; and
- no added fiber in order to provide an energy-dense product.

## Water

In situations that require the distribution of emergency rations to distressed populations, water supplies often will be insufficient or contaminated. Since humans can live only few days without water (Brown, 1947a), ***this report assumes that provision of adequate potable water is the first priority of any emergency operation***. Efforts should also be made to educate indigenous group leaders regarding location of water supplies and water purification (e.g., boiling, iodination). Because of concerns over possible water shortages, the EFP is designed to contribute minimally to osmotic load, while providing essential nutrients and energy to meet the needs of most individuals in emergency situations for a short period of time.

The minimal water requirement for a fasting 70-kg adult, resting in a mild environment, is about 800 ml/day (Gamble, 1947). This is by no means consistent with good health. In the United States, for example, the average adult experiences a water turnover (all sources) of approximately 2,500 ml/day. The lowest volume of fluid required to prevent deterioration provides about 300 ml of urinary output per day. Under low-stress conditions this is equivalent to an intake of about 1,000 ml (Johnson, 1964). According to Gamble (1947) and Marriott (1950), when all water intake ceases, the minimum unavoidable water loss approximates 1,500 ml/day (or about 2 percent of body weight). In a tropical or desert climate, fluid losses may range from 300 ml/h (at rest in shade, 35° C) to 900 ml/h (walking in direct sunlight, 40° C) (Adolph, 1947); this results in total water losses of approximately 3 to 10 percent/8 h exposure for a 70-kg adult. Continuous labor in a desert environment can increase the daily water requirement to 11 L/day, primarily due to sweat losses (Brown, 1947b).

Sustained mental and physical performance are incompatible with the loss of more than 7 to 8 percent of body weight as water (Calloway, 1960). When water losses reach 15 to 25 percent of body weight, it is likely that coma, circulatory failure, and death will occur (Adolph, 1947; Leithead and Lind, 1964). The clinical conditions of heat exhaustion, heat cramps, heat syncope, and heatstroke also are influenced or caused by perturbations of fluid–electrolyte balance (Hubbard et al., 1986).

The state of starvation involves considerable dehydration, regardless of environmental stressors. The actual body water deficit depends on the duration of starvation, water availability, body size, energy intake, dietary composition, work output, and environmental conditions. Infections (e.g., bacterial dysentery) are also common in undernourished individuals, and gastrointestinal illness, with vomiting and diarrhea, obviously increases water and electrolyte losses.

**Carbohydrate Effect on Water Requirement**

When water supplies are insufficient, provision of a minimum of 100 g of carbohydrate in a survival ration is needed (Johnson, 1986). Extensive studies on the composition of survival rations (Calloway, 1960; Gamble, 1947; Grande et al., 1958) have demonstrated that 100 g of carbohydrate constitutes the minimal essential ration amount. This amount of carbohydrate reduced the deficit of body water by lowering the amount of body solutes requiring excretion and by preventing ketosis, thus permitting a reduction in urine volume. The carbohydrate also was essential in maintaining the ability to perform various physical activities by preventing total depletion of glycogen stores, and provides some feeling of satiety.

**Protein Effects on Water Requirement**

Although muscle wasting is common in starvation, inclusion of a large amount of protein in the EFP is contraindicated because it negatively affects water balance. Assuming maximal renal concentration, the excretion of 1 g of urea nitrogen requires 40 to 60 ml of water. This means that the inclusion of 10 g of dietary nitrogen (equivalent to about 63 g of dietary protein) in a 2,100 kcal diet increases the volume of required water by 400 to 600 ml/day. Further, renal concentrating ability is severely compromised in moderate malnutrition (Golden, 2001).

Figure 2-2 depicts the effects of protein and energy content on obligatory urine volume in a multi-level study. The emergency rations tested contained four energy levels (500, 1,000, 1,500, and 2,000 kcal) and four protein levels (0, 7.5, 15, and 30 percent of total calories). In rations that contained 0 and 7.5 percent protein, increasing the caloric content of the ration from 500 to 2,000 kcal did not increase the obligatory urine volume. However, a ration that contained 30 percent protein approximately doubled the obligatory urine volume when the caloric content increased from 500 to 2,000 kcal (Calloway and Spector, 1954).

Based on these calculations and considering the renal dynamics discussed in the previous paragraph, it appears that ***the 2,000 kcal diet was optimal in terms of osmotic load when it contained 7.5 percent protein*** (approximately 40 g of protein). ***The osmotic load created by 15 percent protein appears to be tolerable and this thus becomes the maximum allowable amount.*** Where water availability is of real concern, lower levels of protein should be considered maximal in developing the EFP.

**Salt and Total Dissolved Solids Effects on Water Requirement**

Sodium chloride (NaCl) in emergency rations requires consumption of sufficient water to dilute the added osmotic content to the level found in plasma.

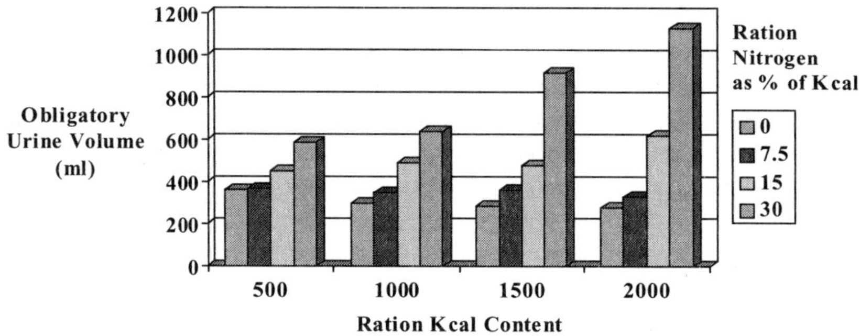


**FIGURE 2-2** Influence of caloric and protein content of emergency rations on urine volume. Excretion of 1 g of urea nitrogen requires 40 to 60 ml of water.

Baker and colleagues (1963) examined the minimal water intake that is needed to dilute various amounts of dietary salt. They overloaded study participants with 11.8, 15.8, and 23.8 g of NaCl for 4 days and 32.8 g of NaCl for 10 days in a 23° C environment. Water was plentiful and was consumed ad libitum. Urinary and fecal excreta eliminated 47 percent of the total water intake and 92 percent of the salt intake. Plasma sodium levels remained constant during the course of metabolic tests, exemplifying the efficacy of renal electrolyte control. Evaluation of water balance indicated that 127 ml of water was required to dilute each gram of NaCl in a 70-kg adult leading a sedentary existence in a mild environment. Thus, the 3 g of Na supplied per 2,100 kcal from the EFP would be equivalent to 7.6 g of NaCl and require 965 ml of water.

Similarly, the human water requirement increases as the total number of osmotically active particles increases in the diet. Because underground wells, reservoirs, and streams contain dozens of minerals, the total dissolved solids (TDS) in water must be considered. Daniels and Layton (1983) have considered the concentrations of TDS in natural water sources. Although they recommend a TDS of 1,000 mg/L for field water supplies, many public drinking water sources in the United States have TDS concentrations exceeding 2,000 mg/L. This indicates that natural field water can have a significant impact on the TDS consumed each day. This should be considered when plans are formulated for the provision of water with emergency rations.

### Summary of Osmotic Load and Water Requirement

There are a variety of nutrients that can increase osmotic load. Some are intracellular osmotic solutes, such as potassium, magnesium, organic phosphates, and protein; some are extracellular osmotic solutes such as sodium and its anions, chloride, and bicarbonate.

Healthy individuals have good renal control of fluid and electrolytes and maintain body equilibrium within a wide range of fluid, sodium, and potassium intakes. However, given the probable circumstances of a population in need of an EFP, body sodium, potassium, and chloride are important components that need to be monitored when a single food source is used to provide all nutrients. Given that various water sources with high levels of solids may significantly increase the osmotic load (Daniels and Layton, 1983), it is important to minimize to the extent possible that contributed by the EFP.

## Electrolytes

### Sodium

Sodium is essential for human health for acid–base balance, body water balance, and nerve function, and it contributes to the palatability of foods. The recommendation for sodium is based on general consumption patterns and available recommendations for maximum intakes (NRC, 1989). Although less than 1 g/day is essential for life, the chronic diarrhea that may be expected in populations requiring the EFP, along with perspiration losses due to elevated ambient temperatures and hard work, increase sodium requirements. Furthermore, additional dietary sodium enhances water retention (Shirreffs et al., 1996) and replaces sodium losses due to diarrhea. Individuals working outdoors with elevated ambient temperatures lose between 2.3 to 3.4 g Na/L of sweat (Costill et al., 1976; Dill et al., 1976). Western dietary guidelines suggest sodium intakes of no more than 2.4 g/day (NRC, 1989). Given that the EFP may be used during periods of sustained physical activity or in high ambient temperatures, the EFP should contain a minimum of 1.3 g/1,000 kcal, which is equivalent to 300 mg/EFP bar. This would provide 1 g of sodium for the 1- to 3-year age group with an average weight of 10 kg and consuming 855 kcal/day (see Tables 2-4 and 2-6). The maximum amount is 1.4 g/1,000 kcal.

### Potassium

Potassium is essential for fluid balance, nerve transmission, and acid–base balance. Similar to sodium, potassium is lost in sweat, feces (diarrhea), and urine, although sweat losses are considered negligible (NRC, 1989). Golden (2001) suggests that a growing child without pre-existing deficiency may need about 1.3 g of potassium/1,000 kcal (2.7 g/2,100 kcal). The recommendation for

**TABLE 2-6** Electrolyte Intake Based on Energy Needs of an Emergency Relief Food Product (EFP)[a]

| Age | Gender | Energy Requirement (kcal/day)[b] | Sodium[c] (g/day) | Potassium[c] (g/day) | Chloride[c] (g/day) |
|---|---|---|---|---|---|
| 7–12 mo[c] | Both | 578 | 0.83 | 0.96 | 1.3 |
| 1–3 yr | Both | 855 | 1.0 | 1.42 | 1.9 |
| 4–8 yr | Both | 1,456 | 2.1 | 2.43 | 3.2 |
| 9–13 yr | Both | 1,693 | 2.4 | 2.82 | 3.7 |
| 14–18 yr | Boys | 2,136 | 3.1 | 3.56 | 4.7 |
| | Girls | 1,931 | 2.8 | 3.22 | 4.2 |
| 19–50 yr | Men | 2,339 | 3.4 | 3.90 | 5.1 |
| | Women | 1,972 | 2.8 | 3.29 | 4.3 |
| 51+ yr | Men | 2,249 | 3.2 | 3.75 | 4.9 |
| | Women | 1,929 | 2.8 | 3.21 | 4.2 |

[a] The EFP contains 1.3 g of sodium, 1.7 g of potassium, and 2.0 g of chloride per 1,000 kcal.
[b] Estimated energy values from Table 2-3.
[c] Based on daily recommendations of no more than 3.0 g of sodium, desirable intake of 3.5 g of potassium, and chloride on an equimolar basis with sodium (NRC, 1989).

the EFP is 1.7 g/1,000 kcal (396 mg/EFP bar), which is given as a desirable intake for adults (NRC, 1989) but much above the minimum requirements, and thus should provide enough to compensate for possible losses due to sweat and mild to moderate diarrhea. The maximum amount is 2.0 g/1,000 kcal (specified content + 20 percent).

### Chloride

Chloride is lost in diarrhea, as well as with vomiting due to its high concentration in gastric juice. Chloride is the principal inorganic anion in extracellular fluid, and is essential for maintaining fluid and electrolyte balance (NRC, 1989). Although chloride deficiency is rarely observed, its loss mirrors sodium loss with the exception of that due to vomiting, so it is also important to ensure adequate intakes of chloride for refugee populations, particularly when consuming a single-source food product. The minimum amount contained in the EFP should be 2.0 g/1,000 kcal to match the sodium content on an equimolar basis. This provides 466 mg of chloride/EFP bar. The maximum amount is 2.2 g/1,000 kcal (specified content + 10 percent). This amount is also equimolar to the sodium level, as recommended by NRC (1989) (see Tables 2-4 and 2-6).

## Summary of Electrolyte Content

Electrolyte content can influence palatability: added sodium in high amounts results in a very salty-tasting product whereas added potassium in high amounts results in a bitter-tasting product. If electrolyte losses are extensive due to chronic severe diarrhea, then therapeutic electrolyte/fluid supplements should be provided (which is beyond the scope of this report).

The nutrient density recommendations for sodium, potassium, and chloride provide additional amounts beyond the recommended intakes for healthy people (NRC, 1989). Because of its bitter taste, food sources should provide the bulk of the potassium.

# Calcium, Phosphorus, and Magnesium

The nutrient content specifications for calcium, phosphorus, and magnesium were derived from the recent evaluation of requirements for these nutrients as part of the DRI process (IOM, 1997). It is assumed that growth stunting is present in the targeted populations (Neumann and Harrison, 1994). There are limited data suggesting that rapid improvement of nutritional status may improve growth, although early stunting is never fully compensated; providing bone-related nutrients early in relief efforts is potentially of benefit. The EFP specifications reflect requirements for children (IOM, 1997a).

Data presented in the DRI report (IOM, 1997a) justify the adequacy of the AI and RDA for calcium and phosphorus, respectively, during adolescence and adulthood as meeting dietary needs during pregnancy and lactation as well. Additional needs are identified during pregnancy for magnesium (IOM, 1997a); however, the individual minimal nutrient density for magnesium (Table 2-4), based on adolescent boys, is actually slightly greater than that derived for pregnancy assuming an additional 200-kcal intake. Thus, additional needs for pregnancy would be met based on the assumption that additional energy (e.g., more EFP bars) would be consumed.

Foods such as soybeans and grains should provide the primary source of these nutrients. However, poor digestibility from plant sources may require some or all of these nutrients to be added to the EFP as direct ingredients in order to provide the specified levels.

## Calcium

Dietary calcium is essential for bone, neuromuscular, and cardiovascular health, as well as for many biochemical functions (IOM, 1997a). During calcium deficiency, the key calcium roles in regulatory proteins are protected at the expense of bone calcium. There is a tight regulation of serum calcium levels through exchange from and to the bone, resorption by the kidney, and absorption from the gastrointestinal tract. Thus, the clinical sign of low calcium status is poor skeletal development, which affects growth, fracture rates, and subsequent rates of osteoporosis.

Bone growth and prevention of osteoporosis are related to chronic intakes of calcium, and there are no data suggesting that suboptimal intakes during a short emergency situation of less than 15 days would have any effect or that supraoptimal intakes during the same short time period would significantly improve bone status. Decreased bone turnover occurs in malnutrition (Branca et al., 1992), but some catch-up (or compensatory) growth is documented with children when adequate overall good nutritional status is restored (Fjeld et al., 1989; Golden, 1994). Although the EFP may provide the only source of nutrients for a very short period of time, the addition of calcium is essential to provide as nutritionally complete a diet as possible.

The minimal nutrient density for calcium is 768 mg/1,000 kcal, which is derived from the AI for children ages 9 through 13 years of 1,300 mg/day (IOM, 1997a). This assumes that these children will consume about 1,700 kcal/day, or 7 to 8 EFP bars (Table 2-3). One bar will contain about 180 mg of calcium.

The source of supplemental calcium used in the EFP should be readily absorbed (certain food sources may decrease the availability of calcium). The role of phytate, oxalic acid, and wheat bran in calcium absorption has been studied (Heaney et al., 1988, 1991; Weaver et al., 1996). Although these compounds decrease calcium absorption, overall there was no significant physiological effect on absorption when provided in a mixed diet (Heaney and Weaver, 1989; Heaney et al., 1990). It is anticipated that cereal grains and legumes will comprise the bulk of the EFP, and thus some sources of phytate will be present. Thus, an increase of 15 percent over the required amount of calcium, 180 mg/EFP bar, is suggested to compensate. The proposed level for calcium may come from supplementation of the food sources to no more than 207 mg/EFP bar (specified content + 15 percent).

The UL for calcium should be considered since the recipient population may have low urinary volumes due to dehydration related to diarrhea and inadequate fluid intakes (Golden, 2001). Urinary loads of calcium must be considered due to calcium interactions with other nutrients that may be deficient in target populations such as iron, zinc, and possibly phosphorus (Golden, 2001). The UL for calcium for adults is 2,500 mg/day based on the adverse effect of milk alkali syndrome seen at higher intake levels (IOM, 1997a). Given the concerns related to renal solute loads discussed earlier, the maximum calcium level should not exceed 885 mg/1,000 kcal.

### Phosphorous

The recommendation for phosphorus is based on its function in growth of soft and bone tissues and replacing phosphorus losses, but not on prevention of a specific sign or symptom of a nutritional deficiency (IOM, 1997a). The phosphorus content of the EFP is set based on the minimal nutrient density of 740 mg/1,000 kcal, which is derived from the RDA of 1,250 mg for boys and girls 9 to 13 years of age based on their estimated energy needs (Table 2-3). One EFP bar of 233 kcal should contain at least 172 mg of phosphorus in an available form. The UL for phosphorus for adults is 4,000 mg based on elevated serum inorganic phosphate levels seen with very high intakes (IOM, 1997a). This level corresponds to a maximum of 1,900 mg of phosphorus/1,000 kcal.

Although potential energy and protein ingredients supply phosphorus for the EFP, the majority of phosphorus from plant foods is in the form of phytic acid, which is less bioavailable (Wyss et al., 1999; Zhou and Erdman, 1995). Furthermore, elevated levels of phytate may impair bioavailability of important trace elements such as zinc. Thus there is a concern about high levels of phytate phosphorus. Method of food processing may also affect mineral availability. Kivisto and colleagues (1986) reported that apparent absorption of magnesium and phosphorus was decreased in an extruded cereal product.

Additional phosphorus to meet the level recommended may be provided by hydrolyzed phytic acid or soluble forms of phosphorus salts such as sodium hypophosphate. The specified range for phosphorus is 740 to 880 mg/1,000 kcal, or 172 to 206 mg/EFP bar (specified content + 20 percent). It is assumed that soybean- and grain-derived ingredients will contribute most of the phosphorus.

## Magnesium

Magnesium is found both in bone (about 50 percent), soft tissue, and extracellular fluid. It is a required cofactor for over 300 enzymes, many of which are involved with energy metabolism and cellular replication. Absorption of magnesium from a typical diet is approximately 50 percent, with fiber decreasing absorption (Kelsay et al., 1979), ostensibly due to its phytate content. The RDA for adults is based on balance studies; the minimal nutrient density for magnesium is based on the requirements of 14- to 18-year-old boys. The recommended amount of magnesium for this subgroup is 190 mg/1,000 kcal based on the energy requirement for this group (Table 2-3) and the RDA (410 mg/d) for magnesium (IOM, 1997a). This amount provides 45 mg of magnesium/EFP bar. A higher level in the EFP is allowed if the source is from food ingredients. The maximum content is 230 mg/1,000 kcal (specified content + 20 percent) in order to ensure that total intake of added magnesium salts is below the adult UL of 350 mg/day. The UL applies only to magnesium salts added to foods, and is a level designed to prevent diarrhea associated with magnesium supplementation. Therefore the maximum amount of added magnesium consumed per day should be below this level, with the magnesium content coming primarily from the

**TABLE 2-7** Recommended Macromineral Content of an Emergency Relief Food Product (EFP)

| Nutrient | RDA or AI[a] for Nutrient Density (mg/d) | Amount/233 kcal Food Bar (mg) | Amount/1,000 kcal of EFP (mg) | Amount/2,100 kcal Ration (mg) |
|---|---|---|---|---|
| Calcium[b] | 1,300 | 180 | 768 | 1,620–1,865 |
| Phosphorus | 1,250 | 172 | 740 | 1,555–1,865 |
| Magnesium | 410 | 45 | 190 | 400[c] |

[a] RDA = recommended dietary allowance, AI = adequate intake.
[b] Calcium recommended intake is an AI rather than an RDA.
[c] The tolerable upper intake level (UL) for magnesium of 350 mg/d applies only to supplemental magnesium, not to magnesium naturally found in foods.

soybean- and grain-derived ingredients. Table 2-7 summarizes the recommended content for calcium, phosphorus, and magnesium in the EFP.

## Trace Elements

### Chromium

Although chromium has been shown to potentiate the action of insulin in vivo and in vitro (IOM, 2001), specific evidence of deficiency in humans has been reported in only a few isolated cases of patients receiving total parenteral nutrition and in malnourished infants who responded to oral doses of chromium chloride (Hopkins and Majaj, 1967). Because of insufficient evidence to set an EAR for chromium, AIs of 35 μg/day and 25 μg/day for men and women 19 through 50 years of age, respectively, were established based on estimated mean energy intakes. Adverse effects have not been demonstrated with excess intakes of chromium per se from food or supplements; consequently, a UL has not been established (IOM, 2001).

Early interest in chromium supplementation to improve growth and glucose utilization in malnutrition has not been applied in current practice (Carter et al., 1968; Gürson and Saner, 1973). The AI values for chromium were based on estimating average amounts of chromium in well-balanced Western diets (which were found to contain on average 13.4 μg/1,000 kcal) (IOM, 2001). Thus a ration containing a minimum of 13.4 μg/1,000 kcal could be expected to meet or exceed the chromium requirement for all healthy persons in a similar population.

This value is higher than the 1.04 μg/1,000 kcal recommended by the Sphere Project as the desirable nutrient density for refugee diets (Sphere Project, 2001). While there is a lack of evidence of deficiency or toxicity and difficulties in analyzing chromium levels in foods, it is important that a single-source food product have some chromium present. It is suggested that the minimum chromium content of the EFP be 13 μg/1,000 kcal (3 μg/EFP bar). The maximum content is not specified in the event that higher amounts are naturally present in the EFP ingredients.

## Copper

Copper deficiency is frequently observed in malnourished populations, particularly in children with protein–energy malnutrition (Ashour et al., 1999; Donma et al., 1990; Squali Houssaïni et al., 1997). Chronic and protracted diarrhea leading to copper depletion has been recognized as a particular concern in infants (Beshgetoor and Hambidge, 1998) and is also a likely risk factor for marginal copper status in adults. The high prevalence of malnutrition and diarrhea characteristic of many groups that will receive the EFP supports the need for adequate copper intake.

Factorial analysis as well as indicators such as plasma copper concentrations, serum ceruloplasmin concentration, erythrocyte superoxide dismutase activity, and platelet copper concentration, are the basis for determining recommended intakes for copper (IOM, 2001).

The minimal nutrient density value for copper was calculated (see Table 2-4) for the limiting subgroup of women 51 years of age and older. Based on the RDA of 900 μg (IOM, 2001), the value required to prevent inadequate intake in almost all individuals in this group would be 470 μg of copper/1,000 kcal. Recognizing the prevalence of malnutrition and diarrhea that often afflicts populations in need of an EFP, the EFP should contain 20 percent above this amount, or 560 μg of copper/1,000 kcal (131 μg/ EFP bar).

Acute liver failure has been demonstrated in individuals consuming large amounts of copper. The UL is 1,000 μg of copper/day for children ages 1 through 3 years (IOM, 2001), more than double the proposed levels for this age group for the EFP (480 μg/855 kcal). The maximum content is 670 μg/1,000 kcal (specified content + 20 percent).

## Iodine

Iodine, a component of thyroxin, is essential for thyroid function and mental development (IOM, 2001). Iodine uptake into the thyroid gland is regulated from the pituitary by thyroid stimulating hormone (TSH). Thus, iodine is part of the regulation of thyroxin production. In iodine deficiency, TSH secretion increases and this may eventually lead to goiter as well as impaired production of thyroid hormones $T_3$ and $T_4$, essential factors for energy regulation and postnatal brain development (Hollowell et al., 1998).

In iodine deficiency, including mild deficiency, dietary iodine supplementation has an immediate impact on thyroid function (Moulopoulos et al., 1988).

Iodine deficiency during pregnancy increases risk of poor fetal mental and physical development, including cretinism. Iodine deficiency disorder (IDD) is considered the most common cause of preventable mental retardation. Iodine deficiency is well established as a nutritional problem worldwide, regardless of refugee status (UNICEF, 2000). In 1999, WHO estimated that 740 million people per year in 130 countries were at risk of IDD, including 50 million who have some degree of IDD-related brain damage. Africa, Southeast Asia, and Asia had the highest concentration of individuals at risk (WHO, 1999b). The use of iodized salt, as well as utilization of iodine for water treatment, is common worldwide. From 1990 to 1998, two-thirds of the households living in IDD-affected countries had access to iodized salt; 20 countries had 90 percent of their households with access to iodized salt.

Iodine is stored in the thyroid gland and deficiency does not occur until that store has been depleted (Clugston and Hetzel, 1994). Aside from inadequate iodine intake, protein–calorie malnutrition also may decrease thyroid iodine levels (Ingenbleek and Malvaux, 1974). Iodine turnover is slow in individuals with adequate iodine status (Fisher and Oddie, 1969).

Iodine is rapidly absorbed in the gastrointestinal tract, and excessive iodine is excreted in the urine. One study suggests that during acute diarrhea associated with protein–calorie malnutrition, iodine may be poorly absorbed (Ingenbleek and Malvaux, 1974). Bioavailability of iodine is generally high, although there are data suggesting inhibition of iodine absorption with soy flour (Shepard et al., 1960). In some populations, linamarin found in cassava may block thyroid uptake of iodine, and there are some data indicating that other water-containing humic substances may block thyroidal iodination.

The most successful method to prevent IDD is iodination of table salt. This is the recommendation of WHO, whose major emphasis is on total prevention of IDD through this practice (WHO, 1999b). WHO recommends that in order to provide 150 μg/day of iodine via iodized salt, iodine concentration in salt at the point of production should be within the range of 20 to 40 mg of iodine (or 34 to 66 mg of potassium iodate) per kg of salt (WHO, 1996a). The EFP should contain iodine as iodized salt although the iodine could also be added as calcium iodide, potassium iodide, or potassium iodate. Dietary studies such as that by Melse-Boonstra and coworkers (2000) indicate that most individuals, regardless of economic, rural, or urban status, purchase salt for cooking.

The minimal nutrient density value for iodine is based on the subgroup of children 1 to 3 years of age and is 105 μg/1,000 kcal. Assuming that iodized table salt will be used in the EFP and provide at least 50 percent of the specified sodium content, the EFP will provide more than adequate levels of iodine to prevent IDD. In the United States, iodized salt contains 194 μg of iodine per g of sodium (Venkatesh Mannar and Dunn, 1995). Thus, if the source of all the sodium in the EFP is from iodized salt, the iodine content of the ration per 1,000 kcal would be approximately 250 μg of iodine. If one assumes that half of the sodium in the EFP may come from nonsalt sources, then the total iodine intake would be half of this, or about 125 μg of iodine/1,000 kcal, which is above the minimum nutrient density needed.

The UL for iodine is based on observations of hypothyroidism, thyroiditis, goiter, and sensitivity reactions (Pennington, 1990). Although little research has been done on refugee populations, iodination of salt in the United States increased the incidence of excessive iodine intake (Hollowell et al., 1998; Pennington, 1990). The UL for children 1 to 3 years of age is 200 μg/day (IOM, 2001), which results in a maximum content of 230 μg/1,000 kcal (specified content + 115 percent). If most of the sodium in the EFP comes from added salt, then it is possible that a mixture of iodized and noniodized salt may be needed to keep the total iodine content below this level. However, if most of the required sodium in the EFP comes from other sources, iodine can be provided in other forms as mentioned previously.

## Iron

Anemia due to iron deficiency represents a major public health problem worldwide. It has been estimated that more than 2 billion people (over 33 percent of the world's population) are iron deficient (INACG, 1999). Young children and women of reproductive age are at greatest risk. Programs to control iron deficiency have been implemented in almost all countries; nevertheless, both anemia and iron deficiency remain endemic among many populations (de Benoist, 2001).

Subclinical and clinical consequences of iron deficiency include impaired physical work performance, developmental delays in infants, cognitive impairment, and adverse pregnancy outcomes (IOM, 2001). Although numerous confounding factors make it difficult to establish a clear relationship, iron deficiency has been reported to be associated with reversible abnormalities of immune function and increased risk of infections (Oppenheimer, 2001; Scrimshaw and SanGiovanni, 1997). A recent conference, organized to evaluate the strength of evidence that iron deficiency causes specific functional outcomes, concluded that there is a significant body of evidence to support a causal relationship among iron deficiency, deficits in work productivity, and child development; and among severe anemia, malnutrition, and increased child mortality. However, causal evidence is lacking or contradictory in support of a relationship between iron deficiency and low birth weight and infectious disease (Stoltzfus, 2001).

The potential adverse effects of excess iron intake also are recognized. High-dose iron supplements have been shown to reduce zinc absorption if both are taken without food; however, this inhibitory effect does not occur if they are consumed with food (IOM, 2001). Similarly, high-dose iron supplements often lead to constipation and other gastrointestinal symptoms when taken without food but usually are not a problem when taken with food (IOM, 2001).

The possibility that high-dose iron supplementation may have adverse effects in individuals with severe malnutrition or infectious diseases also has received attention (Tomkins, 2000). Smith and coworkers (1989) reported an increase in mortality in children with protein–energy malnutrition who received supplements of iron and recommended that iron therapy should not be instituted during the first week of treatment. However, the increase in mortality was not statistically significant and the dosage of iron supplementation was not reported. Based on a comprehensive review of published studies on the relationship between iron and infectious diseases, Oppenheimer (2001) had the following observations of use to health planners: (1) oral iron supplementation has not been shown to cause an increased risk of infection in any age group in nonmalarious countries, (2) oral iron supplementation in malarious regions may carry up to a 50 percent increased risk of clinical malaria if given in therapeutic doses at times of malaria transmission, and (3) oral iron supplementation in therapeutic doses to older immunized children and adults in malarious regions may also carry up to a 50 percent increased risk of other infectious disease. In the studies in malarious regions showing a significant iron-associated increase in risk of nonmalarial infectious morbidity, the dosage of oral iron was 3 mg/kg/day for children 6 months to 6 years of age and 60 mg/day for anemic women.

Review of nine published and four unpublished placebo-controlled, randomized trials of iron supplementation in malarious areas by an expert panel convened by the International Nutritional Anemia Consultative Group led to a consensus statement (INACG, 1999) recommending that oral iron supplementation should continue to be recommended in malarious areas where iron-deficiency anemia is prevalent. It was recognized, however, that present evidence is insufficient to rule out the possibility of an increased risk of malarial illness in some iron-supplemented individuals.

Results of other studies, however, have shown no differences in incidence or severity of conditions such as diarrhea or respiratory infections associated with iron supplementation (Berger et al., 2000; Calder and Jackson, 2000; Oppenheimer, 2001).

It is assumed that as refugees many recipients of the EFP will be iron deficient. Although it is recognized that the deficiency cannot be reversed in 15 days, it is essential that sufficient iron is provided not only to meet basic requirements but also to support the initiation of repletion. The EFP, however, should not contain excess iron, particularly in soluble forms, because excess iron promotes oxidative changes leading to destruction of nutrients such as vitamin C, as well as to the development of rancidity.

Consideration must also be given to the form of iron used in the EFP. Use of iron-EDTA appears to have potential as a fortificant, particularly in diets of low bioavailability. It is less affected by inhibitors of iron absorption and is less likely to cause organoleptic problems, and its efficacy has been demonstrated in several intervention studies (Bothwell, 1999). The possibility of using microencapsulated iron should also be considered (Jackson and Lee, 1991) to minimize problems such as rancidity and inhibit interaction with other nutrients.

Phytic acid, a known inhibitor of iron absorption, will influence the bioavailability of iron from food products (Reddy et al., 2000). Although various approaches are available to reduce the phytate content of the EFP, the most practical approach appears to be fortification of the product at a level of iron that would ensure a sufficient quantity of absorbable iron. Vitamin C has been shown to offset the inhibitory effect of phytate on iron absorption (Hallberg et al., 1989; Siegenberg et al., 1991), thus providing justification for a liberal content of this vitamin in the product (see later section, "Vitamin C").

Factorial modeling was used to calculate recommended intake levels for iron for older infants, children, and adults (IOM, 2001). Using the recommended intake for adult women during their reproductive years (18 mg/day), the minimal nutrient density (Table 2-4) is 9 mg of iron/1,000 kcal. Pregnant women would need higher amounts (12.4 mg/1,000 kcal). The IOM values are based on an assumed bioavailability of 18 percent for children 1 year of age and older, pregnant women during the first trimester, and nonpregnant adults. A mixed protein diet that includes some heme iron is assumed. For children under 1 year of age, for whom the diet will contain little meat and primarily cereals and vegetables, the bioavailability is assumed to be 10 percent; for pregnant women, due to the increased rates of absorption seen during the second and third trimester, bioavailability is assumed to be 25 percent (IOM, 2001).

The provisional recommended daily iron intakes set by the Joint FAO/WHO Expert Consultation on Human Vitamin and Mineral Requirements (FAO/WHO, 2000) for diets having 10 percent iron bioavailability are considerably higher: for girls 10 to 14 years of age, 33 mg (19.5 mg/1,000 kcal); for older adolescents, 31 mg (16 mg/1,000 kcal); and for adult women of reproductive age, 29 mg (14.7 mg/1,000 kcal). To achieve the young adolescent nutrient density, the iron content would need to be doubled to take into account the lower bioavailability.

Since a generous amount of ascorbic acid is included in the EFP, and use of an iron source that is well tolerated and more bioavailable is recommended, the EFP should contain 16.3 mg of iron/1,000 kcal (3.8 mg/EFP bar), assuming 10 percent bioavailablity. This provides the same amount of iron as 9.1 mg/1,000 kcal assuming 18 percent bioavailablility. Given the concern about excess dietary iron and possible adverse effects on immune function, as well as possible food interactions and oxidative changes, the maximum iron content of the EFP is 17.6 mg/1,000 kcal (specified content + 10 percent). A lower iron content may be necessary if this range leads to unacceptable oxidative changes in the product; however, use of encapsulated iron, as mentioned earlier, could help prevent this problem.

## Manganese

Dietary manganese is essential to the action of metalloenzymes involved in the formation of bone and in the metabolism of amino acids, lipids, and carbohydrates. Manganese deficiency has been observed in animals but has only been produced experimentally in humans, thus little data is available related to deficiency in refugee populations. Early signs of inadequate manganese include hypocholsterolemia and a scaling, blistering rash on the upper torso (Friedman et al., 1987; IOM, 2001).

Recommended intakes of manganese are based on median intakes due to insufficient data to determine specific requirements and thus are AIs (IOM, 2001). The minimal nutrient density value is based on the AI for children ages 1 to 3 years (1.2 mg/day) and is 1.4 mg of manganese/1,000 kcal (see Table 2-4). This would provide 0.33 mg of manganese/EFP bar. The maximum content of the EFP is 1.7 mg/1,000 kcal (specified content + 20 percent). Risk of elevated blood manganese concentrations and neurotoxicity are the basis for UL values which range from 2.33 mg/1,000 kcal for children 1 through 3 years of age to 4.70 mg/1,000 kcal for adult males (IOM, 2001).

The level specified for the EFP is much greater than that recommended by the Sphere Project (2001) for a desirable nutrient density of 0.3 μmol/100 kcal (0.2 mg/1,000 kcal) for refugee diets, but it is within the range found in Western diets.

## Selenium

The biological role of selenium is as a component of various selenoproteins. Selenoproteins include five glutathione peroxidases, two deiodinases, several thioredoxin reductases, and selenophosphate synthetase 2 (Behne and Kyriakopoulos, 2001). These proteins are important in supporting immunocompetence and defense against oxidative stress, regulation of thyroid hormone action, and regulation of the redox status of vitamin C and other molecules (IOM, 2000).

Different populations vary greatly in their dietary intake of selenium, largely because the selenium content of plant foods depends on the selenium content of the soil where the food is grown. Meat and fish may be more reliable sources of selenium; however, their content can be influenced by the selenium content in feed sources. Intakes of selenium are particularly low in New Zealand, Finland, and parts of China. Low plasma and hair concentrations of selenium and low plasma glutathione peroxidase activity are common in these countries (Thomson and Robinson, 1996; Varo et al., 1994; Xia et al., 1989). Surveys in other parts of the world suggest that marginal or deficient selenium status may be widespread (Fordyce et al., 2000; Kvicala et al., 1999; Maksimović and Djujić, 1997; Ngo et al., 1997). Low selenium intake leading to severe selenium deficiency is recognized as the major factor contributing to the development of Keshan disease, a cardiomyopathy that occurs primarily in children living in various parts of China (Ge and Yang, 1993). The role of selenium deficiency in Kashin-Beck disease, a degenerative osteoarticular disorder that is endemic to certain low-selenium areas of Tibet, is less clear (IOM, 2000).

Because of the possibility that the selenium status of the population groups receiving the EFP may be marginal or deficient, it can be argued that the ration should provide a generous intake of selenium. Additional support for increasing selenium levels in the EFP is provided by the hypothesized role of selenium in iodine metabolism, oxidative changes associated with protein–energy malnutrition, and viral infections (Ashour et al., 1999; Beck et al., 2001; Contempre et al., 1992; Fechner et al., 2001; Golden, 1998; Levander and Beck, 1999; Ngo et al., 1997; Sive et al., 1993; Tatli et al., 2000; Vanderpas et al., 1990).

The recommended intakes for selenium are based on the criterion of maximizing plasma glutathione peroxidase activity (IOM, 2000) and on data from two intervention studies, one in China and one in New Zealand. Compared to the RDA values (55 μg/day for girls 14 to 18 years old [IOM, 2000]), intakes recommended in a preliminary FAO/WHO (2000) report are considerably lower. Based on the limiting minimal nutrient density (see Table 2-4) of 28 μg of selenium/1,000 kcal (6.5 μg/EFP bar), the minimum amount of selenium should be at this level for the EFP. The maximum content is 34 μg/1,000 kcal (specified content + 20 percent).

Attempts to identify evidence of selenium toxicity in populations living in seleniferous areas of the world have given conflicting results (Reilly, 1996). Residents of seleniferous ranches in South Dakota or Wyoming with intakes as high as 724 μg/day showed no adverse effects associated with their high intakes (Longnecker et al., 1991). In contrast, endemic selenium toxicity occurring in China led to biochemical abnormalities at selenium intakes over 750 μg/day and changes in nails and hair in susceptible individuals at intakes of at least 910 μg/day (Yang et al., 1989). Other signs of chronic toxicity included lesions of the skin, gastrointestinal tract, and nervous system (IOM, 2000).

Hair and nail brittleness and loss are the endpoints on which the UL for selenium is based (IOM, 2000). The maximum nutrient density is 103 μg/1,000 kcal based on the UL for children 4 to 8 years of age. The specified range is well under this maximum. If it is necessary to add selenium to the ration in addition to that provided by the major ingredients, it is recommended that it be in the form of selenomethionine, due to its greater bioavailability compared to selenate and selenite (IOM, 2000). Selenomethionine is the form that has been used in supplementation trials.

## Zinc

Low zinc intakes and marginal or deficient zinc status are found frequently in developing countries, particularly in young children (Zinc Investigators'

Collaborative Group, 2000). However, lack of reliable laboratory biomarkers has made it difficult to accurately estimate the prevalence and severity of zinc deficiency (Hambidge, 2000). Evidence for the existence of inadequate zinc intakes has come largely from zinc supplementation trials (Hotz and Brown, 2001). Consumption of plant-based diets, especially those having a high content of phytic acid, is considered a major factor contributing to zinc deficiency (Gibson et al., 1997; Hambidge et al., 1998).

Zinc intakes recommended by FAO/WHO (2000) vary depending on the estimated bioavailability of dietary zinc. Diets are classified as having high (56 percent), moderate (35 percent), or low (15 percent) zinc bioavailability, based on the dietary content of animal and fish protein, calcium (less or greater than 1 g of calcium/day), and daily molar ratios of phytate to zinc (less than 5, 5 through 15, and greater than 15) (WHO, 1996b).

Zinc bioavailability of the traditional diets consumed by various groups of potential EFP recipients may vary considerably. Using the WHO model, estimates of zinc absorption have ranged from 15 percent for diets in Malawi, Kenya, and Guatemala to 30 percent for diets in Ghana, Guatemala, and Egypt (Gibson and Ferguson, 1998). Thus, if based on dietary zinc content alone, the zinc status of these populations might be expected to differ appreciably; however, other factors such as limited amounts of food and persistent diarrhea may lead to marginal zinc deficiency even in those populations consuming diets low in phytate, a known binder of zinc.

An increasing number of supplementation trials have demonstrated the value of increased zinc intake in promoting linear and ponderal growth in children. For example, a meta-analysis of 25 zinc supplementation trials showed that zinc supplementation had an overall positive effect on change in height (Brown et al., 1998). Subjects in these trials ranged in age from birth to 13 years, with a mean age of 3.6 years. The mean dose of zinc used for supplementation was 14 mg/day (1.5 to 50 mg/day).

A positive effect on growth, however, was not observed in all studies (Friis et al., 1997; Kikafuna et al., 1998). Inconsistent results might be attributed to inclusion of older children whose rate of growth is slower and to the presence of multiple deficiencies that would not be expected to respond to supplementation with a single nutrient (Hotz and Brown, 2001). Some evidence suggests that zinc supplementation may lead to increased activity levels in young children (Sazawal et al., 1996) and improved neuropsychological performance in school-age children (Penland, 2000).

Because zinc deficiency is associated with diarrhea and impaired immune response (IOM, 2001), there is considerable interest in the possible therapeutic or preventive role of zinc in infectious diseases and diarrhea in children in developing countries. A recent study reported a pooled analysis of all available published and unpublished randomized controlled trials of the effect of supplemental zinc in children less than 5 years of age with acute or persistent diarrhea

(Zinc Investigators' Collaborative Group, 2000). In the acute diarrhea trials, zinc-supplemented children had a 15 percent lower probability of continuing diarrhea on a daily basis. In the persistent diarrhea trial analysis, zinc supplementation resulted in a 24 percent lower probability of continuing diarrhea and a 42 percent lower rate of treatment failure or death.

Reports of low dietary intakes of zinc and marginal zinc nutriture in pregnant women are of concern (Fitzgerald et al., 1993; Huddle et al., 1998; Kirksey et al., 1994). Although observational studies have produced strong associations between poor maternal zinc status and various indicators of poor pregnancy outcome, supplementation trials have not produced strong or consistent results in support of dietary zinc supplementation (Caulfield et al., 1998).

The minimal nutrient density value for zinc is 5.2 mg/1,000 kcal, based on boys 14 to 18 years of age (Table 2-4). The RDA for zinc (11 mg/day for adolescent boys) is based on estimates that between 30 and 40 percent of dietary zinc would be absorbed (IOM, 2001). It is doubtful that this level of absorption would occur with the EFP given the plant-based diet with the expected level of phytate. Thus, to cover the potential for reduced absorption due to the type of food ingredients, and due to the presence of gastrointestinal problems in the potential recipient populations, the baseline value is increased by 100 percent, resulting in the specified level of zinc in the EFP of 10.4 mg/1,000 kcal (2.4 mg/EFP bar). This level seems justified on the basis of the demonstrated positive effects of zinc supplementation on growth and in the treatment and prevention of diarrhea in malnourished children

Based on estimates of the zinc content of muscle and changes that occur during malnutrition, Golden (2001) has proposed a level of 13 mg of zinc/1,000 kcal for emergency refugee rations. He concluded that this amount would allow individuals who do not have an initial deficit of zinc to gain at least 5 g/kg of body weight/day even with a diet having low zinc bioavailability. A nutrient density of 13 mg of zinc/1,000 kcal is similar to that in other emergency relief foods such as Corn Soy Blend and Unimix, and lower than that in BP-5 Compact Food or F100 (Golden, 2001). The level chosen for the EFP bar is similar to the desirable nutrient density of 9 mg/1,000 kcal recommended by the Sphere Project (Sphere Project, 2001).

The ULs for zinc, 40 mg/day for adults with lower values for children, are adjusted on a weight basis (IOM, 2001). Other reference values developed as safe upper limits of zinc intake (WHO, 1996b) are higher. The UL for zinc for children ages 1 through 3 years (IOM, 2001) is 7 mg/day, which is less than the proposed level for the EFP for this age group (which totals 8.9 mg/day, based on the estimated energy expenditure for children ages 1 through 3 years).

The UL for zinc is based on the adverse effect of excess zinc on copper status, recognizing that the studies reported were primarily in adults (IOM, 2001). Although this level of zinc in the EFP appears to be of possible concern, the expectation that less will be absorbed also holds true for the UL, and thus a higher amount will in all likelihood not increase the risk that adverse consequences to copper status will occur, particularly when copper is also added to the EFP and the EFP will be fed over a short period of time. However, given the concern about the UL, it is important that the specifications for the EFP be tightly controlled; the maximum content is 11.4 mg/1,000 kcal (specified content + 10 percent).

Additionally, the molar phytate:zinc ratio of the EFP should be less than 10 because higher ratios are associated with suboptimal zinc status (Bindra et al., 1986; Oberleas and Harland, 1981). Consideration needs to be given to the form of zinc added to the EFP. Zinc carbonate and zinc oxide are insoluble and poorly absorbed, whereas zinc sulfate and zinc acetate appear to be better utilized (Allen, 1998) and would be the preferred ingredient.

## Vitamins

### Vitamin A

Vitamin A is required for normal vision, gene expression, reproduction, embryonic development, growth, and immune function (IOM, 2001). Problems associated with vitamin A deficiency reflect these functions. For example, vitamin A deficiency causes blindness as a consequence of xerophthalmia. Vitamin A deficiency is also associated with increased risk for infectious diseases (Underwood and Arthur, 1996). Conversely, infection may contribute to development of vitamin A deficiency as a result of decreased food intake as well as decreased absorption, increased utilization, and possibly increased excretion (Nalubola and Nestel, 1999).

Vitamin A deficiency is a significant public health problem in many parts of the world, especially in Africa and Southeast Asia (WHO, 2001). Clinical vitamin A deficiency affects at least 2.8 million preschool children in more than 60 countries, and it is estimated that subclinical deficiency is a problem in at least 250 million people (Stephenson et al., 2000). School-age children and pregnant women also are affected. An estimated 250,000 to 500,000 children become blind each year as a consequence of severe vitamin A deficiency (WHO, 2001). Importantly, improving the vitamin A status of deficient children, ages 6 months to 5 years, increases their chances of survival, as shown by the meta-analysis of eight studies in which the risk of mortality from diseases such as measles and diarrhea decreased by 23 percent (Beaton et al., 1994).

Many, but not all, studies have shown a beneficial effect of vitamin A supplementation in infectious disease. Meta-analyses by Fawzi and coworkers (1993) and Glasziou and Mackerras (1993) showed a significant reduction in mortality from infectious diseases in children given vitamin A. The value of vitamin A supplementation in improving morbidity, however, is less clear, and results of various studies have been equivocal. Supplementation has been shown to reduce the severity of measles and have a beneficial effect on measles-related pneumonia. However, a beneficial effect on nonmeasles respiratory infections has not been demonstrated (Villamor and Fawzi, 2000). WHO (1999a) has recommended vitamin A supplementation in the management of uncomplicated measles in areas of known deficiency as well as in all cases of complicated measles.

Vitamin A deficiency may be an important factor contributing to poor maternal performance during pregnancy and lactation (Ladipo, 2000; Underwood and Arthur, 1996), as well as growth deficits in children (Hadi et al., 2000; West et al., 1988). Vitamin A is also important in iron metabolism. Impaired mobilization of iron stores was found in the presence of vitamin A deficiency (Lynch, 1997), and a significant increase in mean hemoglobin concentration has been shown in anemic school children given vitamin A supplements (Fishman et al., 2000; Mwanri et al., 2000). Furthermore, the results of a recent study suggest that vitamin A may enhance the absorption of iron from cereal-based meals, possibly by preventing phytic acid from binding iron in the cereals (Layrisse et al., 2000).

The adverse effects of high vitamin A intake are well recognized. Most cases of toxicity have occurred because of high-dose supplements taken over a period of months or years. The possible teratogenicity of high vitamin A levels consumed during the first trimester of pregnancy is of particular concern. However, the threshold at which risk occurs is controversial. Most of the data on birth defects associated with excess vitamin A consumption involve doses equal to or greater than 7,800 μg of preformed vitamin A/day (IOM, 2001), although Rothman and colleagues (1995) showed a significantly increased risk for malformation of cranial structures originating from neural crest cells in the infants of women who consumed more than 4,500 μg/day of preformed vitamin A from food and supplements during the first trimester of pregnancy. The ULs for women 14 through 18 and 19 through 50 years of age are 2,800 and 3,000 μg/day of preformed vitamin A, respectively (IOM, 2001).

The UL for infants is 600 μg/day, based on case reports of infants who developed bulging fontanels as a result of receiving high-dose vitamin A supplements (IOM, 2001). This value is only slightly higher than the AI of 500 μg/day for infants 7 through 12 months of age based on estimated intakes for infants receiving human milk and complementary foods (IOM, 2001). Similarly, the differences between the ULs for children 1 through 8 years of age and their corresponding RDAs are relatively small.

Recommendations for the vitamin A content of diets intended for refugee feeding vary. Beaton (1995) recommended 380 μg of retinol equivalents(RE)/1,000 kcal as a goal for fortification of the total diet for refugee feeding. This amount would be expected to meet the needs of at least 95 percent of

**TABLE 2-8** Vitamin A Content Based on Energy Needs of an Emergency Relief Food Product (EFP)

| Age | Gender | Energy Requirement (kcal/d)[a] | Recommended Dietary Allowance for Vitamin A (μg RAE/day)[b] |
|---|---|---|---|
| 7–12 mo | Both | 578 | 500 (AI) |
| 1–3 yr | Both | 855 | 300 |
| 4–8 yr | Both | 1,456 | 400 |
| 9–13 yr | Both | 1,693 | 600 |
| 14–18 yr | Boys | 2,136 | 900 |
| | Girls | 1,931 | 700 |
| | Girls, pregnant | 2,131 | 750 |
| 19–50 yr | Men | 2,339 | 900 |
| | Women | 1,972 | 700 |
| | Women, pregnant | 2,172 | 770 |
| 51+ yr | Men | 2,249 | 900 |
| | Women | 1,929 | 700 |

[a] Estimated energy values (from Table 2-3).
[b] Taken from IOM, 2001.

individuals and in theory would lead to a 3-month liver reserve. The Sphere Project (2001) suggested that 500 μg RE/day can be used for planning purposes in the initial stages of an emergency. In contrast, Golden (2001) recently recommended that 2,000 μg of retinol/1,000 kcal be added to a ration intended for emergency feeding.

The vitamin A content of diets and products used for refugee relief also varies considerably. For example, the approximate vitamin A content of the BP-5 Compressed Compact Food is 1,025 μg of preformed vitamin A/1,000 kcal (Golden, 2001); Corn/Soy Blend (new), 1,850 μg; and Unimix, 1,635 μg (Beaton, 1995).

The minimal nutrient density value calculated for vitamin A and based on the RDA (900 μg RAE/day [IOM, 2001]) is for boys 14 through 18 years of age (Table 2-4). The value is 420 μg RAE/1,000 kcal. Because the vitamin A status of many of the potential recipients of the EFP may be marginal or deficient and because vitamin A is important in situations involving infectious diseases and diarrhea, the baseline value of 420 μg/1,000 kcal is likely to be too low for many

| Tolerable Upper Intake Level for Preformed Vitamin A (µg/day) | Intake of Vitamin A from EFP[c] Based on Estimated Energy Requirements (µg/day) |
|---|---|
| 600 | 289–578 |
| 600 | 427–855 |
| 900 | 728–1,426 |
| 1,700 | 846–1,693 |
| 2,800 | 1,068–2,136 |
| 2,800 | 966–1,931 |
| 2,800 | 1,066–2,131 |
| | |
| 3,000 | 1,170–2,339 |
| 3,000 | 1,170–2,339 |
| 3,000 | 1,086–2,172 |
| | |
| 3,000 | 1,124–2,249 |
| 3,000 | 964–1,929 |

[c] The EFP contains between 500 and 1,000 µg of preformed vitamin A/1,000 kcal (Table 2-4 and IOM, 2001).

crises. It is recommended that the EFP contain a minimum of 500 µg of preformed vitamin A/1,000 kcal (117 µg/EFP bar). The maximum content is 1,000 µg of preformed vitamin A/1,000 kcal (specified content + 100 percent). Carotenoids possibly present in food ingredients do not contribute to this total due to concern for variable rates of absorption and bioconversion.

Based on assumed energy intakes, the minimum amount exceeds the U.S. and Canadian recommended intakes for all individuals (see Table 2-8). At the maximum amount, intakes of pregnant women would not exceed the UL of 3,000 µg/day of preformed vitamin A (IOM, 2001), although the intake of children 1 through 8 years of age may be 50 percent above their respective UL for the vitamin. However, the UL is designed to represent chronic intake—it is not meant to apply to malnourished individuals who are recipients of fortification or supplementation programs for the prevention and treatment of vitamin A deficiency (IOM, 2001).

If one of the initial activities in a relief program was to give children a high-dose vitamin A supplement (Golden, 2001), it could be argued that the high content of the EFP would not only be unnecessary but also might increase the risk of adverse effects. In view of the sponsors' proposed use of this product such a possibility is unlikely. High-dose supplements are in the range of 60,000 μg of preformed vitamin A administered as a single dose every 4 to 6 months (NRC, 1987); thus the extra amount ingested from food would represent a very small percentage of the total amount given, and consumption of the EFP is recommended for no more than 15 days. It is very important, however, that the content of vitamin A in the EFP be monitored carefully to be within the specifications given.

## Vitamin D

Vitamin D (cholecalciferol) is required for calcium absorption, normal muscle function, and bone growth (IOM, 1997a). Although human requirements can be met with adequate exposure to sunlight (Holick, 1994), it is difficult to monitor and ensure adequate bioconversion. The need for dietary vitamin D for survivability or bone growth for a 15-day period for which the EFP is intended is not clear. However, based on the expectation that the target population is prone to deficiency and a dietary source will enhance the absorption and utilization of calcium, it is recommended that the EFP contain vitamin D. Although not reliably documented, vitamin D deficiency resulting from long periods of wearing full body clothing and living in environments with significant air pollution—especially from dust—is possible.

Clearly, when refugees live close to the equator, vitamin D synthesis is probably occurring when environmental and cultural conditions allow adequate skin exposure to the sun. Because of the complexity of estimating true vitamin D needs in this population, the recommendation for vitamin D content of the EFP is the AI (IOM, 1997a). Populations in need of the EFP can be expected to have a high percentage of individuals under 50 years of age. While the AI for vitamin D is 5 μg of cholecalciferol/day for the adult population 50 years of age and younger, it is 10 μg/day for those between 51 and 70 years of age, and 15 μg/day for those over 70 years of age (IOM, 1997a). The amount of vitamin D for the EFP is proposed to be 5.2 μg/1,000 kcal (1.2 μg/EFP bar), based on the needs for those over 50 years of age; those over 70 years of age were thought to be too small a group within refugee populations to be used as the basis for the vitamin D content of the EFP.

Little information is found concerning the bioavailability of vitamin D in malnourished individuals, so no adjustments were made in the recommendation. The types of ingredients likely to be used in the EFP strongly support the addition of vitamin D as cholecalciferol as there may well be no other dietary source included unless fortified milk solids are used as a protein source. Although dictated by cost, utilization of this form also reduces the potential for toxicity (as compared to $1,25(OH)_2D_3$, the biologically active form of vitamin D). The EFP is not formulated as a therapeutic ration, thus individuals with hepatic or renal disease would need to be treated separately.

The UL for vitamin D is 50 μg of cholecalciferol/day (~24 μg/1,000 kcal), and is based on hypercalcemia at higher levels of intake on a chronic basis (IOM, 1997a). Since the recipient population is likely to have some sun exposure, this limit should be strictly adhered to, as there is a risk in displaced populations—due to dehydration—of compromised urinary function (Briend and Golden, 1993). The maximum content is 5.8 μg/1,000 kcal (specified content + 10 percent).

## Vitamin E

Vitamin E, the primary fat-soluble antioxidant in the body, is essential for proper immune system function and for maintenance of cell membranes. Deficiencies of vitamin E have been reported in malnourished individuals (Golden, 2001). Furthermore, diarrhea and malabsorption are likely to be present in the populations served by the EFP. Absorption of vitamin E is known to be low and varies from 21 to 86 percent depending on the presence of any defects that lead to impaired absorption. Impaired absorption was taken into account in developing the recommended dietary intakes (IOM, 2000). Assuming that a smaller percentage of the dietary vitamin E in the EFP will be absorbed due to possible malabsorption, and recognizing that girls 14 to 18 years of age have the greatest nutrient density need, 20 percent is added to the minimal nutrient density value estimated for this age group (Table 2-4) of 7.8 mg of d-α-tocopherol/1,000 kcal, to provide the amount for the EFP of 9.4 mg/1,000 kcal (2.2 mg/EFP bar). The level of vitamin E should provide adequate antioxidant activity to protect against the oxidation of PUFAs after absorption. Therefore, an additional 6.6 mg of vitamin E is added to protect the maximum amount of PUFA at 10 percent of energy (which is 11 g/1,000 kcal), equivalent to 0.6 mg of vitamin E/g of PUFA.

Since it is recommended that the vitamin E be encapsulated, it is not necessary to provide additional d-α-tocopherol beyond the level specified above to serve as an antioxidant for the PUFA present in the bar. If it is not encapsulated, additional vitamin E or other antioxidants will need to be added to protect against lipid oxidation and subsequent destruction of the vitamin over the shelf life of the EFP.

The required level of d-α-tocopherol (9.4 mg/1,000 kcal) is well below the UL for all groups (1,000 mg total α-tocopherol/day [IOM, 2000]).

## Vitamin K

Vitamin K functions as a cofactor for the blood clotting cascade, and a deficiency is marked by reduced levels of blood clotting factors such as prothrombin factors X, IX, VII, and protein C. Vitamin K is a cofactor for carboxylation of glutamyl residues on proteins to form ϒ-carboxyglutamyl proteins (Gla). Osteocalcin, a Gla protein, is essential for bone formation (IOM, 2001; Olsen, 1994).

Deficiencies of vitamin K are rare in most parts of the world, and there are no data validating vitamin K deficiencies in refugee populations. One study from India showed that breast-fed infants with diarrhea had low levels of prothrombin, suggesting that vitamin K deficiency is independent of antibiotic therapy (Kumar et al., 2001). Children with protein–energy malnutrition also have low prothrombin levels (Hassanein and Tankovsky, 1973), but this deficiency is better treated with an increase in dietary protein than with vitamin K. Besides dietary sources of vitamin K, it has been assumed that the microflora of the gastrointestinal tract synthesize menaquinone. With antibiotic therapy—or in the newborn with a sterile gastrointestinal tract—there is a decrease in vitamin K availability (Kumar et al., 2001). However, the contribution of the bacterially produced vitamin K is unknown (IOM, 2001). Thus, dietary sources are recommended, and vitamin K should be added to the EFP.

Blood clotting is important to survival, especially when there are multiple opportunities for injury due to military-type conflicts as well as the continued movement of many refugee populations. Thus, even a 15-day period of vitamin K supplementation may improve survivability by reducing blood loss due to prolonged clotting time following injury. There are data suggesting some benefit for nursing mothers to consume vitamin K to increase levels in their milk. Due to the limited data, however, the AI is the basis for the vitamin K content of the EFP.

Food composition data suggest that soybean oil (193 μg of vitamin K/100 g) could provide the vitamin K required in the EFP, thereby limiting the need for addition of vitamin K (USDA, 1994). Median and mean intakes of vitamin K have been estimated to be 80 to 120 and 60 to 210 μg/day, respectively, for adult men, the most limiting group (IOM, 2001). Levels that result in deficiency are much lower. Given little concern regarding intake above the AI, the minimum content for the EFP is set at 57 μg/1,000 kcal (14 μg/EFP bar). No maximum level is set as little evidence of adverse effects of overconsumption has been identified, except in those taking prescription anticoagulants.

## Vitamin C

The function of vitamin C in protecting against oxidative stress, its necessity for wound healing, and its likely role in maintaining normal immune function (IOM, 2000) make the vitamin particularly critical for recipients of emergency rations. Vitamin C also is known to enhance the absorption of nonheme iron, which is especially important in populations where iron deficiency is a major nutritional problem, particularly among women and children (IOM, 2000).

Outbreaks of scurvy have been reported in refugee populations during the past three decades, often in populations entirely dependent on emergency food rations found to provide less than 2 mg/day of vitamin C (IOM, 1997b). It is difficult to estimate the actual number of scurvy cases that occur, due partly to lack of adequate surveillance systems in refugee camps, but also because of the frequent existence of multiple deficiencies. Populations under siege or on the move are more likely to encounter problems obtaining fresh fruits and vegetables, the major food sources of vitamin C. Populations in some parts of Africa may have marginal intakes of vitamin C for considerable periods of time before an emergency situation occurs.

The RDA for vitamin C for adults (75 mg/day for women, 90 mg/day for men) is based on the amount needed to maintain near maximal neutrophil ascorbate concentrations with minimal urinary excretion of the vitamin (IOM, 2000). Recommended intakes for children and adolescents are derived from adult values based on body weight. The nutrient density needed to meet the needs of the most limiting group (men over age 50 years; see Table 2-4) is approximately 40 mg/1,000 kcal (IOM, 2000). This level would provide the recommended intakes of vitamin C for healthy adults and exceed those for children.

The vitamin C status of EFP recipients is assumed to be marginal given the likelihood that previous diets were low in fruits and vegetables and the occasional observation of scurvy in some refugee populations. It is also possible that storage in higher heat conditions and possible oxidation may destroy some of the vitamin C present in the EFP. Therefore, it is recommended that the vitamin C content of the EFP be 2.5 times the baseline minimal nutrient density, or 100 mg/1,000 kcal (23.3 mg/EFP bar). This level is similar to that in the BP-5 Compact Food (87 mg/1,000 kcal; Golden, 2001), and slightly lower than that in the USAID Corn/Soy Blend (106 mg/1,000 kcal [IOM, 1997b]).

Given that the ULs for children 1 through 3 and 4 through 8 years of age are 400 mg/day and 650 mg/day, respectively, it is unlikely that levels will be above the UL unless premixing problems arise. Thus, for specifications, the maximum vitamin C content of 200 mg/1,000 kcal is suggested (specified content + 100 percent).

Vitamin C is the most labile of the water-soluble vitamins, and is easily oxidized in the presence of moisture, heat, and light. It is anticipated that significant losses of vitamin C may occur during storage, but the use of an ethylcellulose-encapsulated vitamin C should provide for minimum storage losses (IOM, 1997b). With the overage recommended, adequate vitamin C will be present for the recipient.

### Thiamin

Thiamin is centrally involved in carbohydrate metabolism, nucleic acid and fatty acid synthesis, and membrane and nerve conduction. Anorexia, tiredness, and weight loss are early symptoms of thiamin deficiency; more severe thiamin deficiency leads to cardiovascular and neurological symptoms, including mental changes (Brown, 1990). In adults, beriberi (severe thiamin deficiency) is characterized by varying degrees of peripheral neuropathy and cardiovascular involvement while sustained deficiency leads to death. In young infants (2 to 3 months of age), beriberi is characterized by cardiac symptoms, cyanosis, vomiting, and dyspnea; death can occur within hours of the onset of symptoms (Tanphaichitr, 1994). In young, breast-fed infants, beriberi is due to the thiamin deficiency of the mother. Because ethanol is a thiamin antagonist, chronic and heavy alcohol consumption can lead to thiamin deficiency, manifested as Wernicke-Korsakoff syndrome (Zubaran et al., 1997). The biological half-life of thiamin is approximately 9 to 18 days (Ariaey-Nejad et al., 1970). Therefore, consumption of thiamin-poor diets rapidly leads to poor thiamin status. Thiamin deficiency (unspecified) in individuals with poor initial thiamin status has been noted in refugee situations within 2 weeks (Golden, 2001).

Losses of thiamin during cooking may be considerable due to high temperatures and discarding of cooking water (Kimura et al., 1990). Additionally, thiamin is destroyed by sulfite and chlorite, such as sodium hypochlorite, a disinfectant commonly added to water in refugee camps (Dwivedi and Arnold, 1973; Stammati et al., 1992)

Parasitic infections have been shown to be associated with poorer thiamin status in a sample of young Egyptian men (Hussein et al., 1989). Additionally, thiamin deficiency has been reported among children with severe gastroenteritis (Truswell et al., 1972).

Based on the RDA for the limiting group of children ages 1 to 3 years (0.6 mg/day [IOM, 1998]), the minimal nutrient density necessary to meet recommended intakes is 0.6 mg/1,000 kcal (Table 2-4). The thiamin content of the EFP should be the amount that conservatively meets nutritional requirements under adverse conditions. Due to possible gastrointestinal problems in the target population, and potential destruction of the vitamin due to long-term storage and temperature, the recommended thiamin content is doubled to 1.2 mg/1,000 kcal (0.28 mg/EFP bar). No UL has been set for this nutrient as there are no data on adverse effects from food or supplement intake (IOM, 1998). The maximum content is 1.4 mg/1,000 kcal (specified content + 20 percent).

### Riboflavin

Riboflavin plays a central role in energy metabolism because of its role as the precursor for the coenzymes flavin mononucleotide (FMN) and flavin–adenine dinucleotide (McCormick, 1990, 1994). Both coenzymes function as catalysts for redox reactions, and are involved in numerous metabolic pathways. Riboflavin coenzymes are necessary for the functioning of the electron transport chain. Symptoms of riboflavin deficiency can include painful lesions of the lips and mouth, peripheral nerve dysfunction, and inflammation of the tongue. In general, deficiencies of riboflavin are associated with deficiencies of other nutrients (IOM, 1998).

Significant rates of riboflavin deficiency have been documented in a wide range of populations, including The Gambia (Reddy et al., 1987), northeast Thailand (Pongpaew et al., 1995), Malaysia (Shahar et al., 1999), Guatemala (King et al., 1997), and Zimbabwe (Wacker et al., 2000). In an emergency situation, prior consumption of animal products and green vegetables (major sources of riboflavin) may be limited or absent; therefore riboflavin deficiency can be assumed to be present, particularly if the crisis has been long.

In general, the bioavailability of riboflavin is quite high, although both riboflavin and FMN can form complexes with a variety of substances, including ascorbic acid, tryptophan, zinc, copper, and iron (Jusko and Levy, 1975). Riboflavin is heat stable, and therefore cooking losses are generally minimal, but the vitamin is susceptible to destruction via oxidation and exposure to light.

Diarrhea and other factors that decrease transit time can cause poor absorption (McCormick, 1994). Enhanced losses of riboflavin can occur with catabolic nitrogen losses, and protein–energy malnutrition can be associated with reduced absorption and utilization of riboflavin (McCormick, 1994). Systemic infection, even without gastrointestinal involvement, can increase the riboflavin requirement (McCormick, 1994).

Since riboflavin plays a central role in energy metabolism, the requirement should theoretically be related to energy intake and expenditure. Belko and coworkers (1983, 1984, 1985) examined the effects of dieting and moderate exercise (2.5 to 5 hr/wk) on the riboflavin status of overweight women and found that both activities increased the riboflavin requirement. In The Gambia, the seasonality of riboflavin intake may be associated with changes in energy intake and balance (Bates et al., 1994). Riboflavin requirements may also be increased by a high carbohydrate:fat ratio (Boisvert et al., 1993). Diets of this type are common in developing countries, and are frequently found in refugee situations.

The baseline minimal nutrient density value calculated for riboflavin and based on the RDA (1.3 mg/day [IOM, 1998]) was for boys 14 through 18 years of age (Table 2-4). The value is 0.6 mg/1,000 kcal. Under emergency conditions, riboflavin status may often be compromised by weight loss, heavy exercise, diarrhea, and multiple nutritional deficiencies. Therefore, the baseline value is likely to be too low for many crises. In support of this hypothesis, Bates and coworkers (1989) reported that riboflavin intakes of 1.8 to 2.5 mg/day were required to return a group of Gambian subjects to an acceptable mean erythrocyte glutathione reductase-activity concentration (EGRAC) of 1.3 to 1.4. Furthermore, Belko and coworkers (1985), studying a group of overweight women on low-calorie diets (1,200 to 1,250 kcal/day), found that riboflavin intakes of 1.0 mg/1,000 kcal were associated with elevated EGRAC levels, while a diet containing 1.2 mg/1,000 kcal provided statistically significant improvements in EGRAC values.

The importance of riboflavin in energy metabolism and its potential destruction by heat and light, and the apparent lack of adverse effects of chronic consumption at higher than recommended levels (no UL has been established), suggest that the content of the EFP can be safely doubled to 1.2 mg/1,000 kcal (0.28 mg/EFP bar). This level should be enough to cover any additional requirements due to physical activity and/or diarrhea, and is comparable to the riboflavin content of Unimix (1.1 mg/kcal) and Corn-Soy Blend (1.3 mg/1,000 kcal), although lower than F100 (2.0 mg/1,000 kcal) (Golden 2001). The maximum content is 1.4 mg/1,000 kcal (specified content + 20 percent).

## Niacin

Niacin, through its coenzymes nicotine adenine dinucleotide and nicotine adenine dinucleotide phosphate, plays a central role in energy metabolism, fatty acid and steroid synthesis, DNA repair, and calcium mobilization (Swendseid and Jacob, 1994). Severe niacin deficiency gives rise to the classic deficiency syndrome, pellagra, which is characterized by dermatitis, diarrhea, dementia, and death. Neurological symptoms include apathy, depression, and memory loss. Changes in the digestive track can lead to vomiting, diarrhea, and constipation. Early signs of mild deficiency can include ill-defined gastrointestinal problems, weakness, and lassitude (IOM, 1998). Although the prevalence of mild and marginal deficiencies has not been well documented, rates are likely to be relatively high in some maize- and sorghum-consuming populations (in which niacin deficiency is typically found due to low niacin content along with low levels of tryptophan), particularly during the "hungry season" (the weeks or months when the produce from the previous harvest is fully consumed and the next harvest is not yet ready). The body can convert the amino acid tryptophan to niacin with about 60 mg of tryptophan being needed to produce 1 mg of niacin, although this may vary by as much as 30 percent (IOM, 1998).

Niacin can be obtained either by consumption of preformed niacin or by conversion of tryptophan to niacin. Niacin bioavailability varies according to the form of niacin and the food matrix. In developing countries, many people obtain most of their niacin from grains, legumes, and green leafy vegetables, and by synthesis of niacin from tryptophan. In mature maize, and to a lesser degree in wheat and other cereals, niacin is bound to complex carbohydrates and small peptides and is biologically unavailable (WHO, 2000). Only about 30 percent of niacin in maize is bioavailable; however, heat treatment of maize under alkaline conditions, as is traditionally done in Mexico, greatly increases niacin bioavailability (Carpenter and Lewin, 1985).

Pellagra has often been observed in refugee populations. In 1989 to 1990, an outbreak of pellagra occurred among Mozambican refugees living in Malawi (Malfait et al., 1993). During an 8-month period, nearly 18,000 of 286,000 refugees (incidence = 6.3 percent) were affected (CDC, 1991). Incidence of pellagra

**TABLE 2-9** Recommended Dietary Allowances (RDAs) and Tolerable Upper Intake Levels (ULs) for Niacin

| Age (yr) | RDA (mg of NE[a]/d) | UL[b] (mg/d) | Niacin Intake from the EFP Bar (mg NE/d) |
|---|---|---|---|
| 1–3 | 6 | 10 | 10 |
| 4–8 | 8 | 15 | 16 |
| 9–13 | 12 | 20 | 19 |
| 14–18, boys | 16 | 30 | 24 |
| 14–18, girls | 14 | 30 | 22 |
| Adults, men | 16 | 35 | 26 |
| Adults, women | 14 | 35 | 26 |

[a] NE = niacin equivalents.
[b] As nicotinic acid/niacinamide added to foods or in supplements only (IOM, 1998).
[c] Based on a maximum content of 2.9 mg NE/EFP bar (or 12.4 mg/1,000 kcal).
SOURCE: IOM (1998).

was nearly eight times higher for women than men, but children under 5 years of age were relatively unlikely to be affected. This epidemic was precipitated by a disruption in local groundnut supply, a source of niacin for the population. More recently, an outbreak of pellagra in Angola affected both refugee and local populations (Baquet et al., 2000). Most cases occurred in women (83 percent), with relatively few children under 15 years of age afflicted (18 percent of cases). Other pellagra outbreaks were documented during the 1980s and 1990s in Nepal, Zimbabwe, Angola, Malawi, and Mozambique (WHO, 2000).

Because of the central role of niacin in energy metabolism, niacin requirements bear a theoretical relationship to energy. However, no research has examined the influence of energy expenditure or intake on niacin requirements (IOM, 1998). Additionally, inadequate iron, riboflavin, or vitamin $B_6$ status reduces the efficiency of the conversion of tryptophan to niacin, although the magnitude of these effects has not been established (IOM, 1998).

The limiting subgroup for niacin is boys 14 to 18 years of age (Table 2-4), with a minimal nutrient density needed of 7.5 mg of niacin equivalents (NE)/1,000 kcal. The UL for niacin refers only to nicotinic acid or nicotinamide added to foods or taken as supplements. Thus concern about adverse effects would only arise with the amount of nicotinic acid or nicotinamide added to the EFP.

Because niacin deficiency is likely to be highly prevalent in many refugee populations, the minimal nutrient density is increased by 50 percent to 11.2 mg NE/1,000 kcal (2.6 mg NE/EFP bar). Table 2-9 provides the estimated amount of niacin intakes from the EFP based on the energy intakes estimated in Table 2-3. Given that not all the NE included in the EFP will be as an added ingredient, it is probable that the UL for nicotinic acid/niacinamide will not be exceeded at this level of total niacin intake. However, it is important that the level contained in the EFP be carefully monitored and not be exceeded by more than 10 percent. The maximum content is 12.4 mg/1,000 kcal (specified content + 10 percent).

Golden (2001) has recommended 18 mg/1,000 kcal of niacin. The niacin content of other emergency products ranges from 10 mg/1,000 kcal (F100) to 27 mg/1,000 kcal (Oxford SK8 biscuit). The recommended level for the EFP is within the range of these other recommendations.

### Vitamin $B_6$

Vitamin $B_6$, a group of six compounds of which the pyridoxine forms are the most prevalent in plant-based foods, is important in a wide variety of metabolic processes, including normal protein metabolism and glucose production (IOM, 1998). Adequate vitamin $B_6$ status is also required for optimal conversion of tryptophan to niacin. Hemoglobin synthesis is dependent on adequate vitamin $B_6$ status, and severe deficiency of vitamin $B_6$ can lead to hypochromic, microcytic anemia. Poor vitamin $B_6$ status is associated with compromised cell-mediated immune function. In cases of severe deficiency, infants can suffer convulsions, while symptoms in adults include depression, confusion, irritability, stomatitis, and cheilosis (IOM, 1998).

Little research has been conducted to examine the prevalence of vitamin $B_6$ deficiency in developing countries. In periurban Egypt, 38 percent of 70 women had low vitamin $B_6$ levels in breast milk, and low values were associated with poorer mother–infant interaction (McCullough et al., 1990). In Indonesia, approximately 40 percent of rural third-graders had plasma pyridoxal phosphate values (the most widely used vitamin $B_6$ status index) indicative of deficiency (Setiawan et al., 2000). Vitamin $B_6$ deficiency was observed in 26 percent of young female Chinese textile workers (Ronnenberg et al., 2000). In Europe, the SENECA study found that more than 50 percent of the elderly in some geographical areas had vitamin $B_6$ deficiency (Haller et al., 1991). The results of these studies suggests that pre-existing deficiencies of vitamin $B_6$ can be assumed to be present in refugee populations.

Vitamin $B_6$ is available from a wide range of plant and animal foods. The forms of vitamin $B_6$ in eggs, fish, and poultry are highly bioavailable. Plant pyridoxines are less bioavailable and may decrease absorption of the more bioavailable forms of the vitamin (Gregory, 1998). In developing countries, the principal sources of vitamin $B_6$ are likely to be starchy staples and legumes. Food processing and storage adversely influence the vitamin $B_6$ content of some foods (Leklem, 1996). Vitamin $B_6$ in food is unstable under neutral or alkaline conditions.

Since vitamin $B_6$ is absorbed by a nonsaturable, passive process that occurs primarily in the jejunum, the presence of parasites or diarrhea may have little effect on vitamin $B_6$ absorption, although it has not been well explored. In order to support the role of vitamin $B_6$ in amino acid metabolism, some investigators have proposed an increased requirement for vitamin $B_6$ coincident with increasing protein intake. Several studies have documented a relationship between increased protein intake and decreased vitamin $B_6$ status. However, the precise mathematical relationship remains unclear (IOM, 1998). Several studies have examined the influence of physical activity on vitamin $B_6$ status and metabolism, and have shown little or no relationship (Manore, 2000), although exercise is theoretically linked to increased vitamin $B_6$ requirements.

Based on the RDA of 1.5 mg/day for the limiting subgroup of women 51 years of age and older (IOM, 1998), a minimal nutrient density value was calculated (see Table 2-4). Under the assumptions of the method, the value required to prevent inadequate intake in almost all individuals in this life stage and gender group would be 0.8 mg of vitamin $B_6$/1,000 kcal. Given concern about losses in food processing and storage, the EFP should contain 50 percent more, or 1.2 mg/1,000 kcal (0.28 mg/EFP bar).

Large doses of oral vitamin $B_6$ have been associated with a range of negative outcomes. The UL is 30 g/day as pyridoxine for children ages 1 through 3 years (IOM, 1998), much higher than the proposed level for the EFP. Therefore, adverse effects related to vitamin $B_6$ should not be a problem. The maximum content is 1.4 mg/1,000 kcal (specified content + 20 percent).

### Folate

Folate is a collective term for a family of compounds that are structurally and functionally related to pteroylmonoglutamic acid. Folate is involved physiologically in DNA synthesis, purine synthesis, and amino acid interconversions, including the synthesis of methionine from homocysteine (IOM, 1998). Folate deficiency leads to megaloblastic anemia, elevated homocysteine, increased risk of neural tube defects, and possibly increased risk of other congenital disorders, cancer, and vascular disease (IOM, 1998).

Major sources of folate include green vegetables and legumes. The absorption of food folate requires the conversion of polyglutamyl folates to monoglutamyl forms, which are then absorbed at physiological levels by a saturable transport process (Gregory, 2001). The bioavailability of food folate varies widely by food and may be influenced by processing of the food matrix (Castenmiller et al., 2000; Gregory, 2001). Folate absorption can be adversely effected by unidentified factors in food and by alcohol consumption. Overall, the bioavailability of food folate is estimated at about 50 percent (IOM, 1998). In contrast, synthetic folate in fortified foods is highly bioavailable (~85 percent [IOM, 1998]).

Rates of folate deficiency in developing countries are largely unknown and may be less common than deficiencies of many other micronutrients because of the relatively low cost of legumes and greens, which are major dietary sources.

**TABLE 2-10** Recommended Dietary Allowances (RDAs) and Tolerable Upper Intake Levels (ULs) for Folate

| Age (yr) | RDA (μg DFE[a]/d) | UL[b] (μg synthetic folate/d) | Synthetic Folate Intake[c] (μg/d) |
|---|---|---|---|
| 1–3 | 150 | 300 | 265 |
| 4–8 | 200 | 400 | 452 |
| 9–13 | 300 | 600 | 525 |
| 14–18, boys | 400 | 800 | 662 |
| 14–18, girls | 400 | 800 | 599 |
| Adults, men | 400 | 1,000 | 725 |
| Adults, women | 400 | 1,000 | 611 |

[a] As dietary folate equivalents.
[b] As folate added to foods or in supplements only (IOM, 1998).
[c] Based on a maximum of 80 μg DFE/emergency relief food product bar (or 340 μg/1,000 kcal).
SOURCE: IOM (1998).

However, seasonality, local dietary traditions, or other health conditions may lead to observable rates of deficiency in some populations. In western Venezuela, 91 percent of individuals in a single Bari Indian community were assessed as folate deficient, whereas very little (5 percent) deficiency was observed in a second community (Diez-Ewald et al., 1997). In Malawi, 21 to 34 percent of anemic pregnant women were folate deficient (van den Broek and Letsky, 2000).

Vitamin $B_{12}$ deficiency leads to functional folate deficiency because vitamin $B_{12}$ acts as a cofactor in recycling folate (IOM, 1998). Early research also suggested an adverse effect of zinc deficiency on folate absorption. However, subsequent work has failed to replicate this result (Gregory, 2001).

Using the method previously outlined, the minimal nutrient density value for folate is based on the RDA of 400 μg/day (IOM, 1998) for girls 14 through 18 years of age (Table 2-4). The minimal nutrient density value is 207 μg of dietary folate equivalents (DFE)/1,000 kcal (IOM, 1998). To cover the potential for additional reduced absorption due to gastrointestinal problems, the baseline value is increased by 50 percent and the recommended level of folate for the EFP is 310 μg DFE/1,000 kcal (72 μg DFE/EFP bar).

The UL for folate is 1,000 μg/day for adults, and lower values for children are adjusted on a metabolic weight basis (IOM, 1998) (Table 2-10). The UL for folate is for folate added to foods or taken as supplements only. The UL for children ages 4 through 8 years (IOM, 1998) is 400 μg/day, which is less than the proposed level for the EFP. The UL is based on reports of adverse effects of high levels of folate masking the irreversible neurological damage seen in cases of vitamin $B_{12}$ deficiency. Since some of the folate in the total amount per food bar may be contributed by food sources, it is assumed that this level will not be exceeded. However, given a concern for inadequate mixing, the maximum content is 340 μg DFE/1,000 kcal (specified content + 10 percent). If synthetic folate is used, these values should be divided by 1.6.

### Vitamin $B_{12}$

Vitamin $B_{12}$ is required for methyl transfer to folate; for conversion of homocysteine to methionine; and for synthesis of succinyl CoA, the Krebs cycle intermediate, from L-methylmalonyl CoA. Vitamin $B_{12}$ deficiency can lead to megaloblastic anemia and neuropathy. Neuropsychiatric symptoms can include irritability, fatigue, apathy, and emotional instability (IOM, 1998). Cognitive and neuropsychiatric complications can precede anemia by a considerable period of time. As many as 90 percent of individuals with clinically observable vitamin $B_{12}$ deficiency present neurological complications (IOM, 1998).

Nearly all naturally occurring vitamin $B_{12}$ must be obtained by consumption of animal products, although vitamin $B_{12}$ may be present in small amounts in some plant products via contamination by microorganisms (IOM, 1998). In much of the developing world, animal products are not routinely consumed due to poverty. Some individuals do not consume meat for religious and cultural reasons.

Vitamin $B_{12}$ is efficiently stored in the liver, and losses are minimized in the healthy individual through enterohepatic recirculation. However, because vitamin $B_{12}$ is secreted in the bile as a part of normal digestion, individuals can become deficient due to poor resorption (and absorption) of the vitamin (Stopeck, 2000). *Helicobacter pylori* infection of the gastrointestinal tract may be an important cause of adult vitamin $B_{12}$ deficiency, and treatment of atopic gastritis with antibiotics can be an effective means of reversing $B_{12}$ malabsorption (Kaptan et al., 2000; Suter et al., 1991). In the United States, an estimated 10 to 15 percent of persons aged 60 or older suffer from vitamin $B_{12}$ deficiency, mostly due to poor absorption (Baik and Russell, 1999).

When initial vitamin $B_{12}$ stores are abundant, deficiency due to malabsorption or a vegetarian diet can take years to manifest. However, when low stores are combined with low intake or malabsorption, deficiency occurs more rapidly. In rural Mexico, where consumption of animal products is limited, increased incidence of low levels of vitamin $B_{12}$ in human milk and plasma and decreased holotranscobalamin II have been noted (Allen et al., 1995; Black et al., 1994). High rates of deficiency among children were attributed to maternal malnutrition. In an urban Mexican population, 12 percent of nonpregnant, nonlactating women had low plasma $B_{12}$ values (Casanueva et al., 2000). In Guatemala, 47 percent of lactating women had low plasma $B_{12}$ values, 31 percent of breast milk values were low, and 32 percent of mothers had low holotranscobalamin II values (Casterline et al., 1997). In Malawi, 16 percent of anemic pregnant women were vitamin $B_{12}$ deficient (van den Broek and Letsky, 2000). In Kenya, the vitamin $B_{12}$ content of human milk was very low (Neumann and Harrison, 1994). Epidemiological research in Zimbabwe also suggests that vitamin $B_{12}$ deficiency may be a public health problem in that country (Savage et al., 1994).

The significance of adequate vitamin $B_{12}$ stores is indicated by research on Dutch children who were raised on a macrobiotic diet during the first 6 years of life (Louwman et al., 2000; van Dusseldorp et al., 1999). Subsequently, these children consumed lacto-ovovegetarian or omnivorous diets. However, when assessed during adolescence, vitamin $B_{12}$ status remained low and cognitive function was shown to be impaired. The authors speculated that poor vitamin $B_{12}$ status was the combined effect of low stores from the macrobiotic period and somewhat low subsequent intakes (van Dusseldorp et al., 1999). However, other nutrients were also deficient during the macrobiotic dietary period.

In summary, limited consumption of animal products as a result of poverty concomitant with high rates of diarrhea and gastrointestinal infection due to parasitic and other enteric diseases will likely predispose populations in developing countries to vitamin $B_{12}$ deficiency, and certainly to a lack of stores of the vitamin.

Little information is available on consumption of high levels of vitamin $B_{12}$ from either food or supplements and associated adverse effects; therefore data were inadequate to establish a UL for this vitamin (IOM, 1998).

The minimal nutrient density value for vitamin $B_{12}$ is based on the RDA for girls 14 to 18 years of age (2.4 μg/day [IOM, 1998]), and is 1.2 μg/1,000 kcal (see Table 2-4). However, given the concerns about lack of stores and the probability of a high level of vitamin $B_{12}$ deficiency, higher levels are indicated to ensure that an adequate amount of the nutrient is absorbed and that stores are replenished to the extent possible. Vitamin $B_{12}$ is very stable in foods. Therefore, it is recommended that the baseline value be increased by a factor of 10 to 12 μg/1,000 kcal (2.8 μg/EFP bar). The maximum content is 14.4 μg/1,000 kcal (specified content + 20 percent).

## Pantothenic Acid

Pantothenic acid is required for the synthesis of coenzyme A (CoA), which functions in a broad range of enzymatic processes, many of which involve lipid metabolism (IOM, 1998). CoA is ubiquitously distributed in cells, is required by most forms of life, and is hydrolyzed in the gut to pantothenic acid. Therefore, pantothenic acid can be obtained from a wide range of foods, and pantothenic acid deficiency is thought to be unusual.

Epidemics of deficiency, however, have occurred when food choice was severely restricted. During World War II, prisoners of war in Asia suffered symptoms that were attributed to pantothenic acid deficiency (Plesofsky-Vig, 1999).

More recently, Afghan refugees who were provided white wheat flour without other supplemental food suffered similar symptoms (Golden, 2001). Deficiency can lead to headache, irritability, fatigue, insomnia, nausea and vomiting, hypoglycemia, and paresthesia of the extremities (IOM, 1998).

Absorption of pantothenic acid occurs by active transport at low concentrations, is saturable at higher concentrations, and is passive (Fenstermacher and Rose, 1986). The effects of diarrhea on absorption of pantothenic acid are unknown.

The minimal nutrient density value for pantothenic acid is based on the AI for girls 14 to 18 years of age (5 mg/day [IOM, 1998]) and is 2.6 mg/1,000 kcal (see Table 2-4). The importance of pantothenic acid in energy metabolism, the potential for decreased absorption due to gastrointestinal symptoms or disease, and the lack of reported adverse effects of chronic consumption at higher than recommended levels (no UL has been established) suggest that the content of the EFP can safely be increased by 50 percent to 3.9 mg/1,000 kcal (0.9 mg/EFP bar). The maximum content is 4.7 mg/1,000 kcal (specified content + 20 percent).

### Biotin

Biotin is a cofactor for four adenosine triphosphate-dependent carboxylases (IOM, 1998). This nutrient is necessary for normal cell growth, glucose homeostasis, and DNA synthesis. Biotin deficiency has been shown to be teratogenic in a variety of mammalian species (Mock et al., 1997).

Severe biotin deficiency is rare in the industrialized countries; it occurs due to unusual conditions such as metabolic abnormalities, heavy and sustained intake of avidin from raw egg white, and total parenteral nutrition without biotin supplementation (IOM, 1998). In developing countries, severe protein–energy malnutrition may be accompanied by poor biotin status and impaired carboxylase activity (Velázquez, 1997; Velázquez et al., 1995). Marginal biotin deficiency may be fairly common; a substantial proportion of pregnant women in Iowa exhibited evidence of biotin depletion as pregnancy progressed (Mock et al., 1997). The prevalence of biotin deficiency in both industrialized and developing countries is unknown. A study in rat models has documented an adverse effect of biotin deficiency on *n*-6 PUFA metabolism (Mock, 1990).

Biotin is present in a range of animal and plant foods, but for most foods the precise biotin content and its bioavailability are poorly understood (Said, 1999). Free biotin is nearly 100 percent bioavailable (Zempleni and Mock, 1999). However, much of the biotin in foods is protein-bound and bioavailability is not known (IOM, 1998).

The minimal nutrient density value for biotin is based on the estimated needs of women 51 years of age and older. Based on an AI of 30 μg/day for this group, the baseline value would be 16 μg/1,000 kcal (IOM, 1998). To cover the potential for reduced absorption due to gastrointestinal problems, the minimal nutrient density value is increased by 50 percent to the recommended level for the EFP of 24 μg/1,000 kcal (5.6 μg/EFP bar). The maximum content is 28.8 μg/1,000 kcal (specified content + 20 percent). No UL has been established for biotin; concern about excess intake is unwarranted in this situation.

**Choline**

Choline is involved in the synthesis and release of acetylcholine (a neurotransmitter), and is a precursor of phospholipids and sphingomyelin (important constituents in cell membranes), and also synthesis of the methyl donor, betaine (IOM, 1998). The human body has a limited capacity for de novo choline synthesis and rates of synthesis may not be sufficient to meet the needs of at least some individuals (Zeisel, 2000).

Large amounts of choline are transferred from mother to fetus during pregnancy, and considerable amounts are delivered later to the child via human milk (IOM, 1998). Therefore, adequate maternal intakes of choline are needed to protect the mother against deficiency and to provide the infant with the choline required for normal development. Animal models have demonstrated the importance of adequate choline intake for normal brain development (Blusztajn, 1998). In the rat, choline deficiency adversely influences brain development at two times during growth: during late gestation (12 to 17 days) and postpartum (6 to 30 days) (Jones et al., 1999; Zeisel, 2000). Prenatal effects appear to be permanent (Blusztajn, 1998).

The choline content of foods is poorly characterized, and the bioavailability of many choline-containing compounds in foods is unknown (Zeisel, 2000). However, eggs contain significant amounts of choline, as do liver and peanuts (IOM, 1998).

Free choline is absorbed from the small intestine (Le Kim and Betzing, 1976). The influence of diarrhea, bacterial overgrowth, and parasitic infection on choline absorption is unknown, but it can be assumed to be adverse. No research has been done on the prevalence of choline deficiency in either industrialized or developing countries.

The minimal nutrient density value for choline is based on the AI for the subgroup of men over 50 years of age (550 mg/day [IOM, 1998]), and is 244 mg/1,000 kcal of choline (see Table 2-4). As with other water-soluble vitamins, to cover the potential for reduced absorption due to gastrointestinal problems, the minimal nutrient density value is increased by 50 percent. Therefore, the minimum content is 366 mg/1,000 kcal (85 mg/EFP bar). The maximum content is 439 mg/1,000 kcal (specified content + 20 percent).

## Conclusion

The recommendations for the nutrient content and energy sources contained in this chapter meet the goal of the report: to develop a high-energy, nutrient-dense food product that would be nutritionally adequate for all people 7 months of age and older. The recommendations are designed to provide all known nutrients in quantities to satisfy the needs of the most vulnerable life stage and gender group. In addition, levels of nutrients were frequently increased above the minimal nutrient densities to compensate for poor bioavailability, processing and storage losses, and reduced absorption due to mild diarrhea, infections, or parasites. However, as was described in the beginning of this chapter, the nutritional content is not the highest priority in the design of the ration—in terms of importance, it comes after safety, palatability, ease of delivery, and ease of use.

An additional characteristic that may also be critical is cost. Since this product is intended to be an emergency stop-gap to be used no longer than 15 days while a more permanent food supply line is put in place, if cost is a consideration, it is recommended that food ingredients be analyzed for nutrient content and supplemented only as necessary. It should be assumed that the recommended amounts and sources are considered optimal, but other factors take precedence in the final formulation.

## REFERENCES

Abdallah L, Chabert M, Le Roux B, Louis-Sylvestre J. 1998. Is pleasantness of biscuits and cakes related to their actual or their perceived sugar and fat contents? *Appetite* 30:309–324.

Adolph EF. 1947. Signs and symptoms of desert dehydration. In: Adolph EF, ed. *Physiology of Man in the Desert.* New York: Interscience Publishers. Pp. 226–240.

Allen LH. 1998. Zinc and micronutrient supplements for children. *Am J Clin Nutr* 68:495S–498S.

Allen LH, Backstrand JR, Stanek EJ 3rd, Pelto GH, Chavez A, Molina E, Castillo JB, Mata A. 1992. The interactive effects of dietary quality on the growth and attained size of young Mexican children. *Am J Clin Nutr* 56:353–364.

Allen LH, Rosado JL, Casterline JE, Martinez H, Lopez P, Munoz E, Black AK. 1995. Vitamin $B_{12}$ deficiency and malabsorption are highly prevalent in rural Mexican communities. *Am J Clin Nutr* 62:1013–1019.

Ariaey-Nejad MR, Balaghi M, Baker EM, Sauberlich RE. 1970. Thiamin metabolism in man. *Am J Clin Nutr* 23:764–778.

Ashour MN, Salem SI, El-Gadban HM, Elwan NM, Basu TK. 1999. Antioxidant status in children with protein–energy malnutrition (PEM) living in Cairo, Egypt. *Eur J Clin Nutr* 53:669–673.

Baik HW, Russell RM. 1999. Vitamin $B_{12}$ deficiency in the elderly. *Annu Rev Nutr* 19:357–377.

Baker EM, Plough IC, Allen TH. 1963. Water requirements of men as related to salt intake. *Am J Clin Nutr* 12:394–398.

Baquet S, Wuillaume F, Van Egmond K, Ibanez F. 2000. Pellagra outbreak in Kuito, Angola. *Lancet* 355:1829–1830.

Bates CJ, Powers HJ, Downes R, Brubacher D, Sutcliffe V, Thurnhill A. 1989. Riboflavin status of adolescent vs. elderly Gambian subjects before and during supplementation. *Am J Clin Nutr* 50:825–829.

Bates CJ, Prentice AM, Paul AA. 1994. Seasonal variations in vitamins A, C, riboflavin and folate intake and status of pregnant and lactating women in a rural Gambian community: Some possible implications. *Eur J Clin Nutr* 48:660–668.

Beaton GH. 1995. Fortification of foods for refugee feeding. *Technical Background Report: Derivations and Analyses*. Report to CIDA. Ottawa: Canadian International Development Agency.

Beaton GH, Martorell R, Aronson KA, Edmonston B, McCabe G, Ross AC, Harvey B. 1994. Vitamin A supplementation and child morbidity and mortality in developing countries. *Food Nutr Bull* 15:282–289.

Beck MA, Nelson HK, Shi Q, Van Dael P, Schiffrin EJ, Blum S, Barclay D, Levander OA. 2001. Selenium deficiency increases the pathology of an influenza virus infection. *FASEB J* 15:1481–1483.

Behne D, Kyriakopoulos A. 2001. Mammalian selenium-containing proteins. *Annu Rev Nutr* 21:453–473.

Belko AZ, Obarzanek E, Kalkwarf HJ, Rotter MA, Bogusz S, Miller D, Haas JD, Roe DA. 1983. Effects of exercise on riboflavin requirements of young women. *Am J Clin Nutr* 37:509–517.

Belko AZ, Obarzanek E, Roach R, Rotter M, Urban G, Weinburg S, Roe DA. 1984. Effects of aerobic exercise and weight loss on riboflavin requirements of moderately obese, marginally deficient young women. *Am J Clin Nutr* 40:533–561.

Belko AZ, Meredith MP, Kalkwarf HJ, Obarzanek E, Weinberg S, Roach R, McKeon G, Rose DA. 1985. Effects of exercise on riboflavin requirements: Biological validation in weight reducing women. *Am J Clin Nutr* 41:270–277.

Bemiller JN, Whistler RL. 1996. Carbohydrates. In: Fennema OR, ed. *Food Chemistry*. 3rd ed. New York: Marcel Dekker. Pp. 157–223.

Berger J, Dyck JL, Galan P, Apologan A, Schneider D, Traissac P, Hercberg S. 2000. Effect of daily iron supplementation on iron status, cell-mediated immunity, and incidence of infections in 6–36 month old Togolese children. *Eur J Clin Nutr* 54:29–35.

Beshgetoor D, Hambidge M. 1998. Clinical conditions altering copper metabolism in humans. *Am J Clin Nutr* 67:1017S–1021S.

Bindra GS, Gibson RS, Thompson LU. 1986. [Phytate][calcium]/[zinc] ratios in Asian immigrant lacto-ovo vegetarian diets and their relationship to zinc nutriture. *Nutr Res* 6:475–483.

Black AK, Allen LH, Pelto GH, DeMata MP, Chavez A. 1994. Iron, vitamin $B_{12}$ and folate status in Mexico: Associated factors in men and women and during pregnancy and lactation. *J Nutr* 124:1179–1188.

Blusztajn JK. 1998. Choline, a vital amine. *Science* 281:794–795.

Boisvert WA, Mendoza I, Castañeda C, De Portocarrero L, Solomons NW, Gershoff SN, Russell RM. 1993. Riboflavin requirement of healthy elderly humans and its relationship to macronutrient composition of the diet. *J Nutr* 123:915–925.

Bothwell TH. 1999. Iron fortification with special reference to the role of iron EDTA. *Arch Latinoam Nutr* 49:23S–33S.

Branca F, Robins SP, Ferro-Luzzi A, Golden MHN. 1992. Bone turnover in malnourished children. *Lancet* 340:1493–1496.

Briend A, Golden MHN. 1993. Treatment of severe child malnutrition in refugee camps. *Eur J Clin Nutr* 4:750–754.

Brooks GA, Trimmer JK. 1996. Literature supports the crossover concept. *J Appl Physiol* 80:1073–1074.

Brooks GA, Fahey TP, White TP, Baldwin KM. 2000. *Exercise Physiology. Human Bioenergetics and Its Applications*. Mountain View, CA: Mayfield Publishing. Pp. 723–724.

Brown AH. 1947a. Survival without drinking water in the desert. In: Adolph EF, ed. *Physiology of Man in the Desert*. New York: Interscience Publishers. Pp. 271–279.

Brown AH. 1947b. Water requirements of man in the desert. In: Adolph EF, ed. *Physiology of Man in the Desert*. Pp. 115–135.

Brown KH. 1991. Dietary management of acute childhood diarrhea: Optimal timing of feeding and appropriate use of milks and mixed diets. *J Pediatr* 118:S92–S98.

Brown KH, Lopez de Romana G, Grahan GG, MacLean WC. 1982. Experience with a mixture of wheat-noodles and casein in the initial dietary therapy of infants and young children with protein energy malnutrition or acute diarrhea. *Human Nutr Applied Nutr* 36A:354–366.

Brown KH, Perez F, Gastanaduy AS. 1991. Clinical trial of modified whole milk, lactose-hydrolyzed whole milk, or cereal-milk mixtures for the dietary management of acute childhood diarrhea. *J Pediatr Gastroenterol Nutr* 12:340–350.

Brown KH, Peerson JM, Fontaine O. 1994. Use of nonhuman milks in the dietary management of young children with acute diarrhea: A meta-analysis of clinical trials. *Pediatrics* 93:17–27.

Brown KH, Sanchez-Griñan MI, Perez F, Peerson JM, Ganoza L, Stern JS. 1995. Effects of dietary energy density and feeding frequency on total daily energy intakes of recovering malnourished children. *Am J Clin Nutr* 62:13–18.

Brown KH, Peerson JM, Allen LH. 1998. Effect of zinc supplementation on children's growth: A meta-analysis of intervention trials. *Bibl Nutr Dieta* 54:76–83.

Brown ML. 1990. Thiamin. In: Brown ML, Filer LJ, Guthrie HA, Levander OA, McCormick DB, Olson RE, Steele RD, eds. *Present Knowledge in Nutrition*. 6th ed. Washington, DC: ILSI Press. Pp. 142–145.

Butte NF. 1996. Energy requirements of infants. *Eur J Clin Nutr* 50:S24–S36.

Butte NF, Wong WW, Hopkinson JM, Heinz CJ, Mehta NR, Smith EO. 2000. Energy requirements derived from total energy expenditure and energy deposition during the first 2 y of life. *Am J Clin Nutr* 72:1558–1569.

Cahill GH Jr. 1970. Starvation in man. *N Engl J Med* 282:668–675.

Calder PC, Jackson AA. 2000. Undernutrition, infection and immune function. *Nutr Res Rev* 13:3–29.

Calloway DH. 1960. Nutritional aspects of the all-purpose survival ration. *US Armed Forces Med J* 11:403–417.

Calloway DH, Chenoweth WL. 1973. Utilization of nutrients in milk- and wheat-based diets by men with adequate and reduced abilities to absorb lactose. I. Energy and nitrogen. *Am J Clin Nutr* 26:939–951.

Calloway DH, Spector H. 1954. Nitrogen balance as related to caloric and protein intake in active young men. *Am J Clin Nutr* 2:405–411.

Calloway DH, Murphy S, Balderston J, Receveur O, Lein D, Hudes M. 1992. *Village Nutrition in Egypt, Kenya and Mexico: Looking Across the CRSP Projects*. Final report to the U.S. Agency for International Development. Berkeley, CA: University of California, Berkeley.

Carpenter KJ, Lewin WJ. 1985. A reexamination of the composition of diets associated with Pellagra. *J Nutr* 115:543–552.

Carter JP, Kattab A, Abd-El-Hadi K, Davis JT, el Ghalmy A, Patwardhan VN. 1968. Chromium (III) in hypoglycemia and in impaired glucose utilization in kwashiorkor. *Am J Clin Nutr* 21:195–202.

Casanueva E, Drijanski A, Fernandez-Gaxiola AC, Meza C, Pfeffer F. 2000. Folate deficiency is associated with obesity and anemia in Mexican urban women. *Nutr Res* 20:1389–1394.

Castenmiller JJ, van de Poll CJ, West CE, Brouwer IA, Thomas CM, van Dusseldorp M. 2000. Bioavailability of folate from processed spinach in humans: Effect of food matrix and interaction with carotenoids. *Ann Nutr Metab* 44:163–169.

Casterline JE, Allen LH, Ruel MT. 1997. Vitamin $B_{12}$ deficiency is very prevalent in lactating Guatemalan women and their infants at three months postpartum. *J Nutr* 127:1966–1972.

Caulfield LE, Zavaleta N, Shankar AH, Merialdi M. 1998. Potential contribution of maternal zinc supplementation during pregnancy to maternal and child survival. *Am J Clin Nutr* 68:499S–508S.

CDC (Centers for Disease Control and Prevention). 1990. Health and nutritional profile of refugees—Ethiopia, 1989–1990. *Morb Mortal Wkly Rep* 39:707–709, 715–718.

CDC. 1991. International Notes. Outbreak of pellagra among Mozambican refugees—Malawi, 1990. *Morb Mortal Wkly Rep* 40:209–213.

Chulei R, Xiaofang L, Hongsheng M, Xiulan M, Guizheng L, Gianhong D, DeFrancesco CA, Connor WE. 1995. Milk composition in women from five different regions of China: The great diversity of milk fatty acids. *J Nutr* 125:2993–2998.

Clegg KM. 1960. The availability of lysine in groundnut biscuits used in the treatment of kwashiorkor. *Br J Nutr* 12:325–329.

Clugston GA, Hetzel BS. 1994. Iodine. In: Shils ME, Olson JA, Shike M, eds. *Modern Nutrition in Health and Disease.* 8th ed. Baltimore: Lea & Febiger. Pp. 252–263.

Collins N. 2000. Assessment and treatment of involuntary weight loss and protein–calorie malnutrition. *Adv Skin Wound Care* 13:S4–S10.

Collins S, Myatt M, Golden B. 1998. Dietary treatment of severe malnutrition in adults. *Am J Clin Nutr* 68:193–199.

Contempre B, Duale NL, Dumont JE, Ngo B, Diplock AT, Vanderpas J. 1992. Effect of selenium supplementation on thyroid hormone metabolism in an iodine and selenium deficient population. *Clin Endocrinol* 36:579–583.

Costill DL, Coté R, Fink W. 1976. Muscle water and electrolytes following varied levels of dehydration in man. *J Appl Physiol* 40:6–11.

Crim MC, Munro HN. 1994. Proteins and amino acids. In: Shils ME, Olson JA, Shike M, eds. *Modern Nutrition in Health and Disease*. 8th ed. Baltimore: Lea & Febiger. Pp. 3–35.

Cunnane SC. 1981. Zinc and copper interact antagonistically in the regulation of linoleic acid metabolism. *Prog Lipid Res* 20:601–603.

Dahlin K, Lorenz K. 1993. Protein digestibility of extruded cereal grains. *Food Chem* 48:13–18.

Daniels JI, Layton DW. 1983. *Criteria and Recommendations for Standards for Chloride in Military Field Water Supplies.* Report UCRL-53481. Livermore, CA: Lawrence Livermore National Laboratory.

Day SM, DeHeer DH. 2001. Reversal of the detrimental effects of chronic protein malnutrition on long bone fracture healing. *J Orthop Trauma* 15:47–53.

de Benoist B. 2001. Iron-deficiency anemia: Reexaming the nature and magnitude of the public health problem: Introduction. *J Nutr* 131:564S.

de Bruin NC, Degenhart HJ, Gal S, Westerterp KR, Stijnen T, Visser HK. 1998. Energy utilization and growth in breast-fed and formula-fed infants measured prospectively during the first year of life. *Am J Clin Nutr* 67:885–896.

Decsi T, Molnar D, Koletzko B. 1998. The effect of under- and overnutrition on essential fatty acid metabolism in childhood. *Eur J Clin Nutr* 52:541–548.

De Onis M, Frongillo EA, Blossner M. 2000. Is malnutrition declining? An analysis of changes in levels of child malnutrition since 1980. *Bull World Health Organ* 78:1222–1233.

Diez-Ewald M, Torres-Guerra E, Layrisse M, Leets I, Vizcaino G, Arteaga-Vizcaino M. 1997. Prevalence of anemia, folic acid and vitamin B12 deficiency in two Bari Indian communities from western Venezuela. *Invest Clin* 38:191–201.

Dill DB, Soholt LF, Oddershede IB. 1976. Physiological adjustments of young men to five-hour desert walks. *J Appl Physiol* 40:236–242.

Donma O, Gunbey S, Tas MA, Donma MM. 1990. Zinc, copper, and magnesium concentrations in hair of children from southeastern Turkey. *Biol Trace Elem Res* 24:39–47.

Drewnowski A. 1997. Taste preferences and food intake. *Annu Rev Nutr* 17:237–253.

Drewnowski A, Nordensten K, Dwyer J. 1998. Replacing sugar and fat in cookies: Impact on product quality and preference. *Food Qual Pref* 9:13–20.

Dudley GA, Duvoison MR, Covertinos VA, Buchanan P. 1989. Alterations of the in vivo torque-velocity relationship of human skeletal muscle following 30 days exposure to simulated microgravity. *Avia Space Environ Med* 60:659–663.

Dupont J, White PJ, Carpenter MP, Schaefer EJ, Meydani SN, Elson CE, Woods M, Gorbach SL. 1990. Food uses and health effects of corn oil. *J Am Coll Nutr* 9:438-470.

Dwivedi BK, Arnold RG. 1973. Chemistry of thiamine degradation in food products and model systems: A review. *J Agric Food Chem* 21:54–60.

Enomoto TM, Isichei C, VanderJagt DJ, Fry DE, Glew RH. 1998. Decreased polyunsaturated fatty acids in sickle cell anaemia. *J Trop Pediatr* 44:28–34.

FAO/WHO (Food and Agriculture Organization/World Health Organization). 1989. *Protein Quality Evaluation.* FAO Food and Nutrition Paper 51. Rome: FAO.

FAO/WHO. 1994. *Fats and Oils in Human Nutrition.* FAO Food and Nutrition Paper 57. Rome: FAO.

FAO/WHO. 1998. *Carbohydrates in Human Nutrition.* FAO Food and Nutrition Paper 66. Rome: FAO.

FAO/WHO. 2000. *Preliminary Report on Recommended Nutrient Intakes.* Rome: FAO.

FAO/WHO/UNU (Food and Agriculture Organization/World Health Organization/United Nations University). 1985. *Energy and Protein Requirements*. Technical Report Series No. 724. Geneva: WHO.

Fawzi WW, Chalmers TC, Herrera MG, Mosteller F. 1993. Vitamin A supplementation and child mortality: A meta-analysis. *J Am Med Assoc* 269:898–903.

Fechner A, Böhme C, Gromer S, Funk M, Schirmer R, Becker K. 2001. Antioxidant status and nitric oxide in the malnutrition syndrome kwashiorkor. *Pediatr Res* 49:237–243.

Fenstermacher DK, Rose RC. 1986. Absorption of pantothenic acid in rat and chick intestine. *Am J Physiol* 250:G155–G160.

Fisher DA, Oddie TH. 1969. Thyroid iodine content and turnover in euthyroid subjects: Validity of estimation of thyroid iodine accumulation from short-term clearance studies. *J Clin Endcr* 29:721–727.

Fishman SM, Christian P, West KP. 2000. The role of vitamins in the prevention and control of anaemia. *Public Health Nutr* 3:125–150.

Fitzgerald SL, Gibson RS, Quan de Serrano J, Portocarrero L, Vasquez A, de Zepeda E, Lopez-Palacios CY, Thompson LU, Stephen AM, Solomons NW. 1993. Trace element intakes and dietary phytate/Zn and Ca x phytate/Zn millimolar ratios of periurban Guatemalan women during the third trimester of pregnancy. *Am J Clin Nutr* 57:195–201.

Fjeld CAR, Schoeller DA, Brown KH. 1989. A new model for predicting energy requirements of children during catch-up growth developed using doubly labeled water. *Pediatric Res* 25:503–508.

Fordyce FM, Johnson CC, Navaratna UR, Appleton JD, Dissanayake CB. 2000. Selenium and iodine in soil, rice and drinking water in relation to endemic goitre in Sri Lanka. *Sci Total Environ* 263:127–141.

Friedman BJ, Freeland-Graves JH, Bales CW, Behmardi F, Shorey-Kutschke RL, Willis RA, Crosby JB, Trickett PC, Houston SD. 1987. Manganese balance and clinical observations in young men fed a manganese-deficient diet. *J Nutr* 117:133–143.

Friedman M, Brandon DL. 2001. Nutritional and health benefits of soy proteins. *J Agric Food Chem* 49:1069–1086.

Friis H, Ndhlovu P, Mduluza T, Kaondera K, Sandstrom B, Michaelsen KF, Vennervald BJ, Christensen NO. 1997. The impact of zinc supplementation on growth and body composition: A randomized, controlled trial among rural Zimbabwean school children. *Eur J Clin Nutr* 51:38–45.

Gamble JL. 1947. Physiological information gained from studies on the life raft ration. In: The Harvey Society of New York, eds. *The Harvey Lectures.* Lancaster, PA: The Sciences Press Printing Co. Pp. 247–273.

Ge K, Yang G. 1993. The epidemiology of selenium deficiency in the etiological study of endemic diseases in China. *Am J Clin Nutr* 57:259S–263S.

Gibson RS, Ferguson EL. 1998. Assessment of dietary zinc in a population. *Am J Clin Nutr* 68:430S–434S.

Gibson RS, Donovan UM, Heath A-LM. 1997. Dietary strategies to improve the iron and zinc nutriture of young women following a vegetarian diet. *Plant Foods Hum Nutr* 51:1–16.

Glasziou PP, Mackerras DE. 1993. Vitamin A supplementation in infectious diseases: A meta analysis. *Br Med J* 306:366–370.

Golden MH. 1994. Is complete catch-up possible for stunted malnourished children? *Eur J Clin Nutr* 48:S58–S71.

Golden MH. 1998. Oedematous malnutrition. *Br Med Bull* 54:433–444.

Golden MH. 2001. *The Derivation of the Proposed Nutritional Composition of an Emergency Relief Food for Refugees and Displaced Persons*. Washington, DC: U.S. Agency for International Development.

Golden MH, Waterlow JC, Picou D. 1977. Protein turnover, synthesis and breakdown before and after recovery from protein–energy malnutrition. *Clin Sci Molecular Med* 53:473–477.

Grande F, Taylor HL, Anderson JT, Buskirk E, Keys A. 1958. Water exchange in men on a restricted water intake and a low calorie carbohydrate diet accompanied by physical work. *J Appl Physiol* 12:202–210.

Grange AO, Santosham M, Ayodele AK, Lesi F, Stallings RY, Brown KH. 1994. Evaluation of a maize-cowpea-palm oil diet for the dietary management of Nigerian children with acute, watery diarrhea. *Acta Peadiatr* 83:825–832.

Gregory JF. 1998. Nutritional properties and significance of vitamin glycosides. *Annu Rev Nutr* 18:277–296.

Gregory JF. 2001. Case study: Folate bioavailability. *J Nutr* 131:1376S–1382S.

Grobler-Tanner C. 2001. *A Study of Emergency Relief Foods for Refugees and Displaced Persons*. Washington, DC: U.S. Agency for International Development.

Gürson CT, Saner G. 1973. Effects of chromium supplementation on growth in marasmic protein–calorie malnutrition. *Am J Clin Nutr* 26:988–991.

Hadi H, Stoltzfus RJ, Dibley MJ, Moulton LH, West KP, Kjolhede CL, Sadjimin T. 2000. Vitamin A supplementation selectively improves the linear growth of Indonesian preschool children: Results from a randomized controlled trial. *Am J Clin Nutr* 71:507–513.

Hallberg L, Brunc M, Rossander L. 1989. Iron absorption in man: Ascorbic acid and dose-dependent inhibition by phytate. *Am J Clin Nutr* 49:140–144.

Haller J, Lowik MR, Ferry M, Ferro-Luzzi A. 1991. Nutritional status: Blood vitamins A, E, $B_6$, $B_{12}$, folic acid and carotene. *Eur J Clin Nutr* 45:63–82.

Hambidge M. 2000. Human zinc deficiency. *J Nutr* 130:1344S–1349S.

Hambidge KM, Krebs NF, Miller L. 1998. Evaluation of zinc metabolism with use of stable-isotope techniques: Implications for the assessment of zinc status. *Am J Clin Nutr* 68:410S–413S.

Hassanein EA, Tankovsky I. 1973. Disturbances of coagulation mechanism in protein–calorie malnutrition. *Trop Geog Med* 25:158–162.

Heaney RP, Weaver CM. 1989. Oxalate: Effect on calcium absorbability. *Am J Clin Nutr* 50:830–832.

Heaney RP, Weaver CM, Recker RR. 1988. Calcium absorbability from spinach. *Am J Clin Nutr* 47:707–709.

Heaney RP, Recker RR, Weaver CM. 1990. Absorbability of calcium sources: The limited role of solubility. *Calcif Tissue Int* 46:300–304.

Heaney RP, Weaver CM, Fitzsimmons ML. 1991. Soybean phytate content: Effect on calcium absorption. *Am J Clin Nutr* 53:745–747.

Hirschhorn N. 1980. The treatment of acute diarrhea in children: An historical and physiological perspective. *Am J Clin Nutr* 33:637–644.

Holick MF. 1994. McCollum Award Lecture, 1994: Vitamin D—New horizons for the 21st century. *Am J Clin Nutr* 60:619–630.

Hollowell JG, Staehling NW, Hannon WH, Flanders DW, Gunter ES, Maberly GF, Braverman LE, Pino S, Miller DT, Garbe PL, DeLozier DM, Jackson RJ. 1998. Iodine nutrition in the United States. Trends and public health implications: Iodine excretion data from National Health and Nutrition Examination Surveys I and III. *J Clin Endocrinol Metal* 83:3401–3408.

Holman RT, Johnson SB, Mercuri O, Itarte HJ, Rodrigo MA, De Tomas ME. 1981. Essential fatty acid deficiency in malnourished children. *Am J Clin Nutr* 34:1534–1539.

Hopkins LL Jr, Majaj AS. 1967. Improvements of impaired glucose tolerance by chromium(III) in malnourished infants. In: Kuhnau J, ed. *Proceedings of the Seventh International Congress of Nutrition. Volume 5: Physiology and Biochemistry of Food Components.* London: Pergamon Press. Pp. 721–723.

Hotz C, Brown KH. 2001. Identifying populations at risk of zinc deficiency: The use of supplementation trials. *Nutr Rev* 59:80–88.

Hubbard RW, Armstrong LE, Evans PK, De Luca JP. 1986. Long-term water and salt deficits—A military perspective. In: *Predicting Decrements in Military Performance Due to Inadequate Nutrition.* Washington, DC: National Academy Press. Pp. 29–53.

Huddle JM, Gibson RS, Cullinan TR. 1998. Is zinc a limiting nutrient in the diets of rural pregnant Malawian women? *Br J Nutr* 79:257–65.

Hussein L, Arafah A, Gaafar S. 1989. The vitamin B1 status among young Egyptian males with infection due to parasites. *Int J Vitam Nutr Res* 59:48–51.

INACG (International Nutritional Anemia Consultative Group). 1999. *Consensus Statement: Safety of Iron Supplementation Programs in Malaria-Endemic Regions.* Washington, DC: International Life Sciences Institute Research Foundation.

Ingenbleek Y, Malvaux P. 1974. Iodine balance studies in protein–calorie malnutrition. *Arch Dis Child* 49:305–309.

IOM (Institute of Medicine). 1995a. *Consideration of the Nutrition Components of The Sick Child Initiative*. Washington, DC: National Academy Press.

IOM. 1995b. *Estimated Mean per Capita Energy Requirements for Planning Emergency Food Aid Rations*. Washington, DC: National Academy Press.

IOM. 1997a. *Dietary Reference Intakes for Calcium, Phosphorus, Magnesium, Vitamin D, and Fluoride*. Washington, DC: National Academy Press.

IOM. 1997b. *Vitamin C Fortification of Food Aid Commodities*. Washington, DC: National Academy Press.

IOM. 1998. *Dietary Reference Intakes for Thiamin, Riboflavin, Niacin, Vitamin* $B_6$, *Folate, Vitamin* $B_{12}$, *Pantothenic Acid, Biotin, and Choline*. Washington, DC: National Academy Press.

IOM. 2000. *Dietary Reference Intakes for Vitamin C, Vitamin E, Selenium, and Carotenoids*. Washington, DC: National Academy Press.

IOM. 2001. *Dietary Reference Intakes for Vitamin A, Vitamin K, Arsenic, Boron, Chromium, Copper, Iodine, Iron, Manganese, Molybdenum, Nickel, Silicon, Vanadium, and Zinc*. Washington, DC: National Academy Press.

Ivy JL, Costill DL, Fink WJ, Lower RW. 1979. Influence of caffeine and carbohydrate feeding on endurance performance. *Med Sci Sports Exerc* 11:6–11.

Jackson LS, Lee K. 1991. Microencapsulated iron for food fortification. *J Food Sci* 56:1047–1050.

Jamison E, Hobbs F. 1994. *World Population Profile: 1994*. Report WP/94. Washington, DC: U.S. Bureau of the Census.

James WPT, Schofield EC. 1990. *Human Energy Requirements*. Oxford: Oxford University Press.

Jéquier E. 1999. Response to and range of acceptable fat intake in adults. *Eur J Clin Nutr* 53:S84–S88.

Johnson HL. 1986. Practical military implications of fluid and nutritional imbalances for performance. In: *Predicting Decrements in Military Performance Due to Inadequate Nutrition*. Washington, DC: National Academy Press. Pp. 55–67.

Johnson RE. 1964. Water and osmotic economy on survival rations. *J Am Diet Assoc* 45:124–129.

Jones JP, Meck WH, Williams CL, Wilson WA, Swartzwelder HS. 1999. Choline availability to the developing rat fetus alters adult hippocampal long-term potentiation. *Brain Res Dev* 118:159–167.

Jusko WJ, Levy G. 1975. Absorption, protein binding, and elimination of riboflavin. In: Rivlin RS, ed. *Riboflavin*. New York: Plenum Press. Pp. 99–152.

Kalra V, Grover JK, Ahuja GK, Rathi S, Gulati S, Kalra N. 2001. Vitamin E administration and reversal of neurological deficits in protein–energy malnutrition. *J Trop Pediatr* 47:39–45.

Kaptan K, Beyan C, Ural AU, Cetin T, Avcu F, Gulsen M, Finci R, Yalcin A. 2000. *Helicobacter pylori*—Is it a novel causative agent in vitamin $B_{12}$ deficiency? *Arch Intern Med* 160:1349–1353.

Kelsay JL, Behall KM, Prather ES. 1979. Effect of fiber from fruits and vegetables on metabolic responses of human subjects, II. Calcium, magnesium, iron, and silicon balances. *Am J Clin Nutr* 32:1876–1880.

Kikafuna JK, Walker AF, Allan EF, Tumwine JK. 1998. Effect of zinc supplementation on growth and body composition of Uganda preschool children: A randomized, controlled, intervention trial. *Am J Clin Nutr* 68:1261–1266.

Kimura M, Itokawa Y, Fujiwara M. 1990. Cooking losses of thiamin in food and its nutritional significance. *J Nutr Sci Vitaminol (Tokyo)* 36:S17–S24.

King JE, Mazariegos M, Valdez C, Castaneda C, Solomons NW. 1997. Nutritional status indicators and their interpretations in rural Guatemalan elderly: A study in San Pedro Ayampuc. *Am J Clin Nutr* 66:795–802.

Kirksey A, Wachs TD, Yunis F, Srinath U, Rahmanifar A, McCabe GP, Galal OM, Harrison GG, Jerome NW. 1994. Relation of maternal zinc nutriture to pregnancy outcome and infant development in an Egyptian village. *Am J Clin Nutr* 60:782–792.

Kivisto B, Andersson H, Cederblad G, Sandberg AS, Sandstrom B. 1986. Extrusion cooking of a high-fibre cereal product. 2. Effects on apparent absorption of zinc, iron, calcium, magnesium and phosphorus in humans. *Br J Nutr* 55:255–260.

Koletzko B. 1999. Response to and range of acceptable fat intakes in infants and children. *Eur J Clin Nutr* 53:S78–S83.

Koletzko B, Abiodun PO, Laryea MD, Bremer HJ. 1986. Fatty acid composition of plasma lipids in Nigerian children with protein–energy malnutrition. *Eur J Pediatr* 145:109–115.

Koletzko B, Thiel I, Abiodun PO. 1992. The fatty acid composition of human milk in Europe and Africa. *J Pediatr* 120:S62–S70

Kumar R, Marwaha N, Marwaha RK, Garewal G. 2001. Vitamin K deficiency in diarrhoea. *Indian J Pediatr* 68:235–238.

Kvicala J, Zamrazil V, Jiranek V. 1999. Characterization of selenium status of inhabitants in the region Usti nad Orlici, Czech Republic by INAA of blood serum and hair and fluorimetric analysis of urine. *Biol Trace Elem Res* 71:31–39.

Ladipo OA. 2000. Nutrition in pregnancy: Mineral and vitamin supplements. *Am J Clin Nutr* 72:280S–290S.

Laryea MD, Leichsenring M, Mrotzek M, el-Amin EO, el Kharib AO, Ahmed HM, Bremer HJ. 1995. Fatty acid composition of the milk of well-nourished Sudanese women. *Int J Food Sci Nutr* 46:205–214.

Layrisse M, Garcia-Casal MN, Solano L, Baron MA, Arguello F, Llovera D, Ramirez J, Leets I, Tropper E. 2000. New property of vitamin A and beta-carotene on human iron absorption: Effect on phytate and polyphenols as inhibitors of iron absorption. *Arch Latinoam Nutr* 50:243–248.

Leichsenring M, Sutterlin N, Less S, Baumann K, Anninos A, Becker K. 1995. Polyunsaturated fatty acids in erythrocyte and plasma lipids of children with severe protein–energy malnutrition. *Acta Paediatr* 84:516–520.

Leithead CS, Lind AR. 1964. *Heat Stress and Heat Disorders.* Philadelphia: Davis. P. 304.

Le Kim D, Betzing H. 1976. Intestinal absorption of polyunsaturated phosphatidylcholine in the rat. *Hoppe Seylers Z Physiol Chem* 357:1321–1331.

Leklem JE. 1996. Vitamin B-6. In: Ziegler EE, Filer LJ, eds. *Present Knowledge in Nutrition*. 7th ed. Washington, DC: ILSI Press. Pp. 174–183.

Levander OA, Beck MA. 1999. Selenium and viral virulence. *Br Med Bull* 55:528–533.

Longnecker MP, Taylor PR, Levander OA, Howe SM, Veillon C, McAdam PA, Patterson KY, Holden JM, Stampfer MJ, Morris JS, Willett WC. 1991. Selenium in diet, blood, and toenails in relation to human health in a seleniferous area. *Am J Clin Nutr* 53:1288–1294.

Lopez-Pedrosa JM, Torres MI, Fernandez MI, Rios A, Gil A. 1998. Severe malnutrition alters lipid composition and fatty acid profile of small intestine in newborn piglets. *J Nutr* 128:224–233.

Louwman MWJ, van Dusseldorp M, van de Vijver F, Thomas CMG, Schneede J, Ueland PM, Refsum H, van Staveren WA. 2000. Signs of impaired cognitive function in adolescents with marginal cobalamin status. *Am J Clin Nutr* 72:762–769.

Lynch SR. 1997. Interaction of iron with other nutrients. *Nutr Rev* 55:102–110.

Maksimović ZJ, Djujić I. 1997. Selenium deficiency in Serbia and possible effects on health. *Biomed Environ Sci* 10:300–306.

Malfait P, Moren A, Dillon JC, Brodel A, Begkoyian G, Etchegorry MG, Malenga G, Hakewill P. 1993. An outbreak of pellagra related to changes in dietary niacin among Mozambique refugees in Malawi. *Int J Epidemiol* 22:504–511.

Manore MM. 2000. Effect of physical activity on thiamin, riboflavin, and vitamin B-6 requirements. *Am J Clin Nutr* 72:598S–606S.

Marin MC, De Tomas ME, Mercuri O, Fernandez A, de Serres CT. 1991. Interrelationship between protein–energy malnutrition and essential fatty acid deficiency in nursing infants. *Am J Clin Nutr* 53:466–468

Marin MC, De Tomas ME, Serres C, Mercuri O. 1995. Protein–energy malnutrition during gestation and lactation in rats affects growth rate, brain development and essential fatty acid metabolism. *J Nutr* 125:1017–1024.

Marriott HL. 1950. *Water and Salt Depletion.* Springfield, IL: Thomas.

Martorell R, Habicht JP. 1986. Growth in early childhood in developing countries. In: Falkner F, Tanner JM, eds. *Human Growth: A Comprehensive*

*Treatise. Volume 3: Methodology Ecological, Genetic, and Nutritional Effects on Growth.* New York: Plenum Press. Pp. 241–262.

McCormick DB. 1990. Riboflavin. In: Brown ML, Filer LJ, Guthrie HA, Levander OA, McCormick DB, Olson RE, Steele RD, eds. *Present Knowledge in Nutrition.* 6th ed. Washington, DC: ILSI Press. Pp 146–154.

McCormick DB. 1994. Riboflavin. In: Shils ME, Olson JA, Shike M, eds. *Modern Nutrition in Health and Disease.* 8th ed. Baltimore: Lea & Febiger. Pp. 366–375.

McCullough AL, Kirksey A, Wachs TD, McCabe GP, Bassily NS, Bishry Z, Galal OM, Harrison GG, Jerome NW. 1990. Vitamin $B_6$ status of Egyptian mothers: Relation to infant behavior and maternal–infant interactions. *Am J Clin Nutr* 51:1067–1074.

Melse-Boonstra A, Pee S, Halati ME, Kosen SM, Muhilal S, Bloem M. 2000. The potential of various foods to serve as a carrier for micronutrient fortification, data from remote areas in Indonesia. *Eur J Clin Nutr* 54:822–827.

Mock DM. 1990. Evidence for a pathogenic role of omega 6 polyunsaturated fatty acid in the cutaneous manifestations of biotin deficiency. *J Pediatr Gastroenterol Nutr* 10:222–229.

Mock DM, Stadler DD, Statton SL, Mock NI. 1997. Biotin status assessed longitudinally in pregnant women. *J Nutr* 127:710–716.

Moulopoulos DS, Mantzox JM, Souvatzoglou A, Piperingos GD, Karaiskos KS, Makriyannis D, Stontouris J, Moulopoulos SD. 1988. The relation of serum $T_4$ and TSH with the urinary iodine excretion. *J Endoc Invest* 11:437–439.

Mwanri L, Worsley A, Ryan P, Masika J. 2000. Supplemental vitamin A improves anemia and growth in anemic school children in Tanzania. *J Nutr* 130:2691–2696.

Nalubola R, Nestel P. 1999. *The Effect of Vitamin A Nutriture on Health: A Review.* Washington, DC: ILSI Press. P. 10.

Neumann CG, Harrison GG. 1994. Onset and evolution of stunting in infants and children. Examples from the Human Nutrition Collaborative Research Support Program. Kenya and Egypt studies. *Eur J Clin Nutr* 48:S90–S102.

Neumann C, McDonald MA, Sigman M, Bwibo N, Marquardt M. 1991. Relationships between morbidity and development in mildly to moderately malnourished Kenyan toddlers. *Pediatrics* 88:934–942.

Ngo DB, Dikassa L, Okitolonda W, Kashala TD, Gervy C, Dumont J, Vanovervelt N, Contempre B, Diplock AT, Peach S, Vanderpas J. 1997. Selenium status in pregnant women of a rural population (Zaire) in relation to iodine deficiency. *Trop Med Int Health* 2:572–581.

NRC (National Research Council). 1987. *Vitamin A Supplementation. Methodologies for Field Trials.* Washington, DC: National Academy Press.

NRC. 1989. *Recommended Dietary Allowances.* 10th ed. Washington, DC: National Academy Press.

Oberleas D, Harland BF. 1981. Phytate content of foods: Effect on dietary zinc bioavailability. *J Am Diet Assoc* 79:433–436.

Okolo SN, VanderJagt TJ, Vu T, VanderJagt TA, VanderJagt DJ, Okonji M, Huang YS, Chuang LT, Onwuanaku C, Glew RH. 2000. The fatty acid composition of human milk in northern Nigeria. *J Hum Lact* 16:28–35.

Olsen RE. 1994. Vitamin K. In: Shils ME, Olson JA, Shike M, eds. *Modern Nutrition in Health and Disease.* 8th ed. Baltimore: Lea & Febiger. Pp. 342–358.

Oppenheimer SJ. 2001. Iron and its relation to immunity and infectious disease. *J Nutr* 131:616S–635S.

Penland JG. 2000. Behavioral data and methodology issues in studies of zinc nutrition in humans. *J Nutr* 130:361S–364S.

Pennington JA. 1990. A review of iodine toxicity reports. *J Am Diet Assoc* 90:1571–1581.

Penny ME, Brown KH. 1992. Lactose feeding during persistent diarrhoea. *Acta Paediatr* 381:133–138.

Plesofsky-Vig N. 1999. Pantothenic acid. In: Shils ME, Olson JA, Shike M, Ross CA, eds. *Modern Nutrition in Health and Disease.* 9th ed. Baltimore: Williams & Wilkins. Pp. 423–432.

Pongpaew P, Saowakontha S, Schelp FP, Rojsathaporn K, Phonrat B, Vudhivai N, Supawan V, Intarakhao C, Mahaweeravat U, Lumbiganon P, Sanchaisurya P, Migasena P. 1995. Vitamins B1, B2 and B6 during the course of pregnancy of rural and urban women in northeast Thailand. *Int J Vitam Nutr Res* 65:111–116.

Prentice AM, Goldberg GR. 2000. Energy adaptations in human pregnancy: Limits and long-term consequences. *Am J Clin Nutr* 71:1226S–1232S.

Prentice AM, Paul AA. 2000. Fat and energy needs of children in developing countries. *Am J Clin Nutr* 72:1253S–1265S.

Prentice AM, Lucas A, Vasquez-Velasquez L, Davies PS, Whitehead RG. 1988. Are current dietary guidelines for young children a prescription for overfeeding? *Lancet* 2:1066–1069.

Prentice AM, Spaaij CJ, Goldberg GR, Poppitt SD, van Raaij JM, Totton M, Swann D, Black AE. 1996. Energy requirements of pregnant and lactating women. *Eur J Clin Nutr* 50:S82–S110.

Reddy VA, Bates CJ, Goh SG, Rowland MG, Greenwood AM, Greenwood B, Paul AA. 1987. Riboflavin, folate and vitamin C status of Gambian women during pregnancy: A comparison between urban and rural communities. *Tran R Soc Trop Med Hyg* 81:1033–1037.

Reddy MB, Hurrell RF, Cook JD. 2000. Estimation of nonheme-iron bioavailability from meal composition. *Am J Clin Nutr* 71:937–943.

Reilly C. 1996. *Selenium in Food and Health*. London: Blackie Academic and Professional. Pp. 110–117.

Rice AL, Sacco L, Hyder A, Black RE. 2000. Malnutrition as an underlying cause of childhood deaths associated with infectious diseases in developing countries. *Bull World Health Organ* 78:1207–1221.

Riley SA, Marsh MN. 1998. Maldigestion and malabsorption. In: Feldman M, Sleisenger MH, Scharschmidt BF, eds. *Sleisenger & Fordtran's Gastrointestinal Disease: Pathophysiology, Diagnosis, Management*. 6th ed. Philadelphia: Saunders. Pp. 1053–1054.

Rocquelin G, Tapsoba S, Dop MC, Mbemba F, Traissac P, Martin-Prevel Y. 1998. Lipid content and essential fatty acid (EFA) composition of mature Congolese breast milk are influenced by mothers' nutritional status: Impact on infants' EFA supply. *Eur J Clin Nutr* 52:164–171.

Rolls BJ. 2000. The role of energy density in the overconsumption of fat. *J Nutr* 130:268S–271S.

Rolls BJ, Bell EA. 1999. Intake of fat and carbohydrate: Role of energy density. *Eur J Clin Nutr* 53:S166–S173.

Ronnenberg AG, Goldman MB, Aitken IW, Xu X. 2000. Anemia and deficiencies of folate and vitamin B-6 are common and vary with season in Chinese women of childbearing age. *J Nutr* 130:2703–2710.

Rothman KJ, Moore LL, Singer MR, Nguygen UDT, Mannino S, Milunsky B. 1995. Teratogenicity of high vitamin A intake. *N Engl J Med* 333:1369–1373.

Said HM. 1999. Biotin bioavailability and estimated average requirement: Why bother? *Am J Clin Nutr* 69:352–353.

Saltzman E, Dallal GE, Roberts SB. 1997. Effect of high-fat and low-fat diets on voluntary energy intake and substrate oxidation: Studies in identical twins consuming diets matched for energy density, fiber and palatability. *Am J Clin Nutr* 66:1332–1339.

Sanchez-Griñan MI, Peerson JM, Brown KH. 1992. Effect of dietary energy density on total ad-libitum energy consumption by recovering malnourished children. *Eur J Clin Nutr* 46:197–204.

Santosham M, Brown KH, Sack RB. 1987. Oral rehydration therapy and dietary therapy for acute childhood diarrhea. *Pediatr Rev* 8:273–278.

Savage D, Gangaidzo I, Lindebaum J, Kiire C, Kukiibi JM, Moyo A, Gwanzura C, Mudenge B, Bennie A, Sitima J. 1994. Vitamin $B_{12}$ deficiency is the primary cause of megaloblastic anaemia in Zimbabwe. *Br J Haematol* 86:844–850.

Sazawal S, Bentley M, Black RE, Dhingra P, George S, Bhan MK. 1996. Effect of zinc supplementation on observed activity in low socioeconomic Indian preschool children. *Pediatrics* 98:1132–1137.

Schmeits BL, Okolo SN, VanderJagt DJ, Huang YS, Chuang LT, Mata JR, Tsin AA, Glew RH. 1999. Content of lipid nutrients in the milk of Fulani women. *J Hum Lact* 15:113–120.

Scrimshaw NS, Murray EB. 1988. The acceptability of milk and milk products in populations with a high prevalence of lactose intolerance. *Am J Clin Nutr* 48:1083–1159.

Scrimshaw NS, SanGiovanni JP. 1997. Synergism of nutrition, infection, and immunity: An overview. *Am J Clin Nutr* 66:464S–477S.

Setiawan B, Giraud DW, Driskell JA. 2000. Vitamin $B_6$ inadequacy is prevalent in rural and urban Indonesian children. *J Nutr* 130:553–558.

Shahar S, Earland J, Powers HJ, Rahman SA. 1999. Nutritional status of rural elderly Malays: Dietary and biochemical findings. *Int J Vitam Nutr Res* 69:277–284.

Shepard TH, Pyne GE, Kirschvink JF, McLean CM. 1960. Soybean goiter, report of three cases. *N Eng J Med* 262:1099–1103.

Sherman WM. 1983. Carbohydrates, muscle glycogen, and muscle glycogen supercompensation. In: Williams MH, ed. *Ergogenic Aids in Sport*. Champaign, IL: Human Kinetics. Pp. 3–26.

Shirreffs SM, Taylor AJ, Leiper JB, Maughan RJ. 1996. Post-exercise rehydration in man: Effects of volume consumed and drink sodium content. *Med Sci Sports Exerc* 28:1260–1271.

Siegenberg D, Baynes RD, Bothwell TH, Macfarlane BJ, Lamparelli RD, Car NG, MacPhail P, Schmidt U, Tal A, Mayet F. 1991. Ascorbic acid prevents the dose-dependent inhibitory effects of polyphenols and phytates on nonheme-iron absorption. *Am J Clin Nutr* 53:537–541.

Sive AA, Subotzky EF, Malan H, Dempster WS, Heese HD. 1993. Red blood cell antioxidant enzyme concentrations in kwashiorkor and marasmus. *Ann Trop Paediatr* 13:33–38.

Smit EN, Dijkstra JM, Schnater TA, Seerat E, Muskiet FA, Boersma ER. 1997. Effects of malnutrition on the erythrocyte fatty acid composition and plasma vitamin E levels of Pakistani children. *Acta Paediatr* 86:690–695.

Smith IF, Taiwo O, Golden MHN. 1989. Plant protein rehabilitation diets and iron supplementation of the protein–energy malnourished child. *Eur J Clin Nutr* 43:763–768.

Sphere Project. 2001. *The Humanitarian Charter and Minimum Standards in Disaster Response*. Herndon, VA: Stylus Publishing LLC.

Squali Houssaïni FZ, Iraqi MR, Arnaud J, Richard MJ, Favier A. 1997. Trace elements and protein–calorie malnutrition in the Fes area (Morocco). *Biomed Pharmacother* 51:349–351.

Stammati A, Zanetti C, Pizzoferrato L, Quattrucci E, Tranquilli GB. 1992. In vitro model for the evaluation of toxicity and antinutritional effects of sulphites. *Food Addit Contam* 9:551–560.

Stein TP. 1995. Protein metabolism. In: Torosian MH, ed. *Hospital Based Nutrition: Science and Principles of Practice*. New York: Pergamon Press. Pp. 73–87.

Stephenson LS, Latham MC, Ottesen EA. 2000. Global malnutrition. *Parasitol* 121:S5–S22.

Stoltzfus RJ. 2001. Iron-deficiency anemia: Reexaming the nature and magnitude of the public health problem. Summary: Implications for research and programs. *J Nutr* 131:697S–701S.

Stopeck A. 2000. Links between *Helicobacter pylori* infection, cobalamin deficiency, and pernicious anemia. *Arch Intern Med* 160:1229–1230.

Stubbs RJ, Habron CG, Prentice AM. 1996. Covert manipulation of the dietary fat to carbohydrate ratio of isoenergetically dense diets: Effect on food intake in feeding men ad libitum. *Int J Obes* 20:651–660.

Suarez FL, Savaiano DA, Levitt MD. 1995. A comparison of symptoms after the consumption of milk or lactose-hydrolyzed milk by people with self-reported severe lactose intolerance. *N Engl J Med* 333:1–4.

Suter PM, Golner BB, Goldin BR, Morrow FD, Russell RM. 1991. Reversal of protein-bound vitamin $B_{12}$ malabsorption with antibiotics in atrophic gastritis. *Gastroenterol* 101:1039–1045.

Swendseid ME, Jacob RA. 1994. Niacin. In: Shils ME, Olson JA, Shike M, eds. *Modern Nutrition in Health and Disease*. 8th ed. Baltimore: Lea & Febiger. Pp. 376–382.

Tagle MA. 1988. Changes in the patterns of food consumption in Latin America. *Arch Latinoam Nutr* 38:750–765.

Tanphaichitr V. 1994. Thiamin. In: Shils ME, Olson JA, Shike M, eds. *Modern Nutrition in Health and Disease.* 8th ed. Baltimore: Lea & Febiger. Pp. 351–365.

Tatli MM, Vural H, Koc A, Kosecik M, Atas A. 2000. Altered anti-oxidant status and increased lipid peroxidation in marasmic children. *Pediatr Int* 42:289–292.

Thomson CD, Robinson MF. 1996. The changing selenium status of New Zealand residents. *Eur J Clin Nutr* 50:107–114.

Tomkins A. 2000. Malnutrition, morbidity and mortality in children and their mothers. *Proc Nutr Soc* 59:135–146.

Torun B, Davies PS, Livingstone MB, Paolisso M, Sackett R, Spurr GB. 1996. Energy requirements and dietary energy recommendations for children and adolescents 1 to 18 years old. *Eur J Clin Nutr* 50:S37–S80.

Truswell AS, Hansen JD, Konno T. 1972. Thiamin deficiency in children with severe gastro-enteritis. *S Afr Med J* 46:2083–2084.

Uauy R, Mena P, Valenzuela A. 1999. Essential fatty acids as determinants of lipid requirements in infants, children and adults. *Eur J Clin Nutr* 53:S66–S77.

Underwood BA, Arthur P. 1996. The contribution of vitamin A to public health. *FASEB J* 10:1040–1048.

UNHCR (United Nations High Commissioner for Refugees). 2000. *Handbook for Emergencies.* 2nd ed. Geneva: UNHCR. Pp. 220–227.

UNICEF (United Nations Children's Fund). 2000. *Ending Iodine Deficiency Forever*. New York: UNICEF.

UN Subcommittee on Nutrition. 2001. *Report on the Nutrition Situation of Refugees and Displaced Populations*. RNIS 32 & 33. Geneva: UN.

USDA (U.S. Department of Agriculture). 1994. *Provisional Table on the Vitamin K Content of Foods*. HNIS/PT-104. Washington, DC: U.S. Government Printing Office.

Valk EE, Hornstra G. 2000. Relationship between vitamin E requirement and polyunsaturated fatty acid intake in man: A review. *Int J Vitam Nutr Res* 70:31–42.

van den Broek NR, Letsky EA. 2000. Etiology of anemia in pregnancy in south Malawi. *Am J Clin Nutr* 72:247S–256S.

VanderJagt DJ, Arndt CD, Okolo SN, Huang YS, Chuang LT, Glew RH. 2000. Fatty acid composition of the milk lipids of Fulani women and the serum phospholipids of their exclusively breast-fed infants. *Early Hum Dev* 60:73–87.

Vanderpas JB, Contempre B, Duale NL, Goossens W, Bebe N, Thorpe R, Ntambue K, Dumont J, Thilly CH, Diplock AT. 1990. Iodine and selenium deficiency associated with cretinism in northern Zaire. *Am J Clin Nutr* 52:1087–1093.

van Dusseldorp M, Schneede J, Ueland PM, Thomas CMG, de Boer E, van Staveren WA. 1999. Risk of persistent cobalamin deficiency in adolescents fed a macrobiotic diet in early life. *Am J Clin Nutr* 69:664–667.

van Stratum P, Lussenberg RN, van Wezel LA, Vergroesen AJ, Cremer HD. 1978. The effect of dietary carbohydrate:fat ratio on energy intake by adult women. *Am J Clin Nutr* 31:206–212.

Varo P, Alfthan G, Huttunen JK, Aro A. 1994. Nationwide selenium supplementation in Finland—Effects on diet, blood and tissue levels, and health. In: Burk RF, ed. *Selenium in Biology and Human Health*. New York: Springer-Verlag. Pp. 199–218.

Velázquez A. 1997. Biotin deficiency in protein–energy malnutrition: Implications for nutritional homeostasis and individuality. *Nutrition* 13:991–992.

Velázquez A, Tercin M, Baez A, Gutierrez J, Rodriquez R. 1995. Biotin supplementation affects lymphocyte carboxylases and plasma biotin in severe protein–energy malnutrition. *Am J Clin Nutr* 61:385–391.

Venkatesh Mannar MG, Dunn JT. 1995. Choice and dose of iodine compound for salt iodization. In: *Salt Iodization for the Elimination of Iodine Deficiency*. The Netherlands: International Council for Control of Iodine Deficiency Disorders.

Villamor E, Fawzi WW. 2000. Vitamin A supplementation: Implications for morbidity and mortality in children. *J Infect Dis* 182:S122–S133.

Wacker J, Fruhauf J, Schulz M, Chiwora FM, Volz J, Becker K. 2000. Riboflavin deficiency and preeclampsia. *Obstet Gynecol* 96:38–44.

Weaver CM, Heaney RP, Teegarden D, Hinders SM. 1996. Wheat bran abolishes the inverse relationship between calcium load size and absorption fraction in women. *J Nutr* 126:303–307.

West KP, Djunaedi E, Pandji A, Kusdiono, Tarwotjo I, Sommer A. 1988. Vitamin A supplementation and growth: A randomized community trial. *Am J Clin Nutr* 48:1257–1264.

WHO (World Health Organization). 1996a. *Recommended Iodine Levels in Salt and Guidelines for Monitoring Their Adequacy and Effectiveness.* WHO/Nut/96.13. Geneva: WHO.

WHO. 1996b. *Trace Elements in Human Health and Nutrition.* Geneva: WHO. Pp. 72–104.

WHO. 1999a. *Guidelines for Epidemic Preparedness and Response to Measles Outbreaks.* WHO/CDC/CSR/ISR/99.1 Geneva: WHO.

WHO. 1999b. *World Health Organization Sets out to Eliminate Iodine Deficiency Disorder.* Press Release WHA/17. WHO, Geneva. May 25.

WHO. 2000. *Pellagra and Its Prevention and Control in Major Emergencies.* WHO/NHD/00.10. Geneva: WHO.

WHO. 2001. *Combating Vitamin A Deficiency.* Online. Available at http://www.who.int/nut/vad.htm. Accessed January 31, 2002.

Wyss M, Brugger R, Kronenberger A, Rémy R, Fimbel R, Oesterhelt G, Lehmann M, van Loon APGM. 1999. Biochemical characterization of fungal phytases (*myo*-inositol hexakisphosphat phosphohydrolases): Catalytic properties. *Appl Environ Microbiol* 65:367–373.

Xia YM, Hill KE, Burk RF. 1989. Biochemical studies of a selenium-deficient population in China: Measurement of selenium, glutathione peroxidase, and other oxidant defense indices in blood. *J Nutr* 199:1318–1326.

Xiang M, Lei S, Li T, Zetterstrom R. 1999. Composition of long chain polyunsaturated fatty acids in human milk and growth of young infants in rural areas of northern China. *Acta Paediatr* 88:126–131.

Yang G-Q, Yin S, Zhou R-H, Gu L, Yan B, Liu Y, Liu Y. 1989. Studies of safe maximal daily dietary Se-intake in a seleniferous area of China. II. Relation between Se-intake and the manifestation of clinical signs and certain biochemical alterations in blood and urine. *J Trace Elem Electrolytes Health Dis* 3:123–130.

Young H, Jaspars S. 1995. Nutrition, disease and death in times of famine. *Disasters* 19:94–109.

Young H, Fellow P, Mitchell J. 1985. Development of a high energy biscuit for use as a food supplement in disaster relief. *J Food Technol* 20:689–695.

Young H, Owen M, Clark J. 1988. A comparison of biscuits used in emergency relief feeding programmes in Ethiopia and eastern Sudan—1985/86. *Eur J Clin Nutr* 42:261–271.

Zeisel SH. 2000. Choline: An essential nutrient for humans. *Nutrition* 16:669–671.

Zempleni J, Mock DM. 1999. Advanced analyses of biotin metabolites in body fluids allows a more accurate measurement of biotin bioavailability and metabolism in humans. *J Nutr* 129:494S–497S.

Zhou JR, Erdman JW Jr. 1995. Phytic acid in health and disease. *Crit Rev Food Sci Nutr* 35:495–508.

Zinc Investigators' Collaborative Group. 2000. Therapeutic effects of oral zinc in acute and persistent diarrhea in children in developing countries: Pooled analysis of randomized controlled trials. *Am J Clin Nutr* 72:1516–1522.

Zubaran C, Fernandes JG, Rodnight R. 1997. Wernicke-Korsakoff syndrome. *Postgrad Med J* 73:27–31.

# 3

# Processing and Packaging of the Emergency Food Product

Developing energy-dense nutritional foods that can be packaged and stored for extended periods of time in environments that vary from arctic to tropical presents a challenge to the processor. In an emergency situation these products must also meet the nutritional needs of all age groups from infants to adults, and be sufficiently palatable to be consumed for up to two weeks as the sole food. Nutrient profiles for an emergency food product (EFP) can and have been developed (see Chapter 2), but the required useful life of the product will be met only through careful consideration and selection of ingredients, processing techniques, and packaging materials. Key considerations include microbiological and chemical safety, dispersability, and ease of use.

## DESIRABLE CHARACTERISTICS OF AN EMERGENCY RELIEF FOOD PRODUCT

The use of a few nutrient-dense products in a variety of emergencies by relief organizations such as the United Nations High Commissioner for Refugees, the World Food Programme of the United Nations, and the International Committee of the Red Cross and Red Crescent, has resulted in anecdotal information about the desirable characteristics of such foods. These characteristics should be taken into consideration during prototype development in order to develop a superior EFP. Historically, some of the most important emergency relief food products available in Europe, particularly the most successful one—the Norwegian BP-5—were not developed with food relief in mind. They were intended to be rations stowed in lifeboats for use in the event of passengers and crews having to abandon ship. Nevertheless, their use in the field during diverse emergencies, such as the Ethiopia and Eastern Sudan famine of 1985 to 1986 and the more recent Balkans conflicts, have permitted an evaluation of their efficacy from the standpoint of nutrition, acceptability, ease of delivery, and some practical aspects such as potential for diversion seldom discussed in refereed publications. The following sections provide some aspects that representatives from various relief organizations urged be considered in developing specifications for the EFP.

### Packaging the EFP for Airdrop or Surface Delivery

Considering that the EFP is for use at the onset of emergencies, when infrastructure destruction and security considerations make it impossible to run feeding centers, the EFP should be available in a packaging modality amenable to low-altitude airdrop as well as delivery on land. There have been attempts to configure EFPs in ways that facilitate air delivery without damaging the product upon impact on the ground or hurting the intended recipients. Such packaging must also allow for dissemination of the product over a wide area so that it may reach many people. (Past experience indicates that concentrating the drop in the form of parachuted pallets, for example, contributed to hoarding, thus defeating the primary objective of ample distribution of the food relief, and also contributed to its diversion to unintended uses).

### Packaging the EFP to Discourage Diversion

Information provided by relief organizations indicate that the high energy content of some EFPs, the density of nutrients in them, and the ease with which they may be carried has resulted in these products being collected by military combatants in emergency situations involving armed conflict. Biscuit-type EFPs are easily diverted to become military rations in emergencies involving armed conflict to the detriment of and even at a risk to the intended civilian recipients. The diversion is facilitated when the shape and size of the unit makes it easy to fit into the side pockets of military wear; rectangular, thin presentations seem to be best suited for this purpose. In addition, the use of eye-catching, glittery, space-age packaging materials encourages such diversion. It has been, therefore, the consensus among representatives of several relief agencies that the shape and size of the outside package of a successful EFP should be uncomfortable to carry in military pockets and should be made of nonlustrous materials. Furthermore, separation of the ration into smaller portions that cannot easily be rewrapped after opening also discourages diversion while aiding in apportioning the ration among children and adults.

## Packaging to Facilitate Distribution and Consumption of the EFP and Reuse of its Secondary Package

Based on information from relief organizations, other anecdotal considerations for a superior EFP are the size of the unit and the potential for reuse of the secondary package. It is important that the size of the total unit and its breakdown into meal portions are designed so that adults can apportion it to individual sittings. Meal-size portions should be scored to facilitate partitioning them for children.

It is also important that the primary and secondary packages be able to serve additional uses in emergency situations. For example, a combustible primary package for emergency rations has found use in various emergencies as fuel for cooking. The secondary package may also be put to good use by recipients. For example, tin cans used to package emergency rations have been used as containers for water, as storage boxes, and even as metal shingles for building roofs after being pounded flat. In addition, from the technical standpoint, this type of secondary packaging might be very helpful in maintaining the integrity of the EFP against impact and pressure damage, insect and rodent attack, and other environmental challenges during transport, storage, and delivery. Therefore, the secondary package for the EFP should be designed such that it could afford secondary uses to the recipients.

## Characteristics of Similar Ration Products

Conventional and novel technologies were considered for manufacturing the EFP. Combining some of these technologies may be the best approach to optimize the stability of the product and preserve its nutritional and sensory qualities. Dehydration, infusion, compression, and cold extrusion are some examples of processing technologies to be considered. These processes have been tested by the U.S. Army to obtain calorie-dense rations (Briggs et al., 1986; Schulz et al., 1992). A caloric density of 1.1 kcal/cc can be obtained using dehydration and compression. Higher caloric densities (up to 5 to 6 kcal/cc) are also possible using extrusion. The U.S. Air Force General Purpose (GP) Survival Packet ration for aircraft and life rafts, in turn, includes a variety of compressed bars such as a shortbread bar, a chocolate chip bar, a granola bar, and a corn flake cereal bar. The GP is designed to be consumed for periods of less than 5 consecutive days and contains approximately 100 g of carbohydrate and a low protein level (< 8 percent of calories) to counteract the effects of starvation and to conserve body water. This ration provides 1,447 kcal with 18 g of protein (5 percent of calories), 202 g of carbohydrate (56 percent of calories), and 64 g of fat (39 percent of calories). Its storage requirement is 5 years at 80° F and 1 month at 140° F (SBCOMM, 2001a).

The Meal Ready-to-Eat, Individual (MRE) is the standard military ration developed to support the individual soldier in all the U.S. Armed Forces (Army, Air Force, Navy, and Marine Corps). The MRE replaced the C Ration in the early 1980s and has since been continuously updated. It is designed to serve as the sole source of food for up to 10 days in a field environment, until group rations are available. Its use has in many situations been for longer—up to 145 days were reported during the Gulf War in 1993. Feedback from Operations Desert Shield and Desert Storm suggested that soldiers would consume more if their preferences were taken into account (IOM, 1993).

Improvements have focused on revising items to make the rations more acceptable and to expand variety (SBCOMM, 2001b). For example, the MRE bread is a pouch bread (Natick Research, Development, and Engineering Center, 1993) that contains glycerol, sucrose esters, lipids, and sorbic acid to extend shelf life up to 3 years, and has received high hedonic ratings (Hallberg and Chinachoti, 1992). This is now in every MRE ration. The average equilibrium pH and water activity of this bread are 5.0 and 0.86, respectively. The bread is further preserved by controlling oxygen content and initial microbial load (Hallberg et al., 1990; Powers and Berkowitz, 1990).

In an investigation to develop a high-energy biscuit for use as an EFP in disaster relief, low-moisture (3.5 percent) biscuits were prepared using a traditional baking method, with formulation and processing strategies as the means to control caloric density and sensory quality (Young et al., 1985). The products were highly acceptable to sensory panels made up of children both in England and India. This shows that traditional processing methods—perhaps in combination with some of the novel MRE technologies described above—can be used to produce baked EFPs such as biscuits having desirable sensory and nutritional qualities and long shelf life.

## Role of Water Activity, Water Mobility, and Water Content in Packaged Food Products

Three aspects of water are important to consider in describing a food system: water activity ($a_w$), water mobility, and water content. Water activity is defined as the ratio of partial pressure of water in the product over that of pure water at the same temperature. The concept of $a_w$ was first put forward in the early 1950s, as a means of explaining the availability of water for chemical and biological reactions. It has been a useful tool in the food industry for many years and it is particularly useful when dealing with intermediate and high moisture biological systems (Ruan and Chen, 1998; Taoukis et al., 1988). The rate-limiting step in a chemical reaction is frequently associated with the mobility of water and its ability to participate in those reactions. At low $a_w$, the binding of water (monolayer moisture) to components of the system makes it unavailable as a solvent. As $a_w$ increases, water exists in multilayers and is more mobile.

Solvation and reactant mobility increase, so biological and chemical changes occur. This classic general relationship between moisture content, $a_w$, and reaction rate was characterized over 30 years ago (Labuza, 1971).

Water activity is used to predict the stability of food systems and quality changes likely to occur. However, in the past 10 years there have been numerous papers pointing out the limitations of the concept (Frank, 1991; Ruan and Chen, 1998; Slade and Levine, 1991). There are practical and theoretical concerns because $a_w$ measurement assumes that the food system is at equilibrium, a condition where the partial vapor pressure above the food system is the same as that of the water within it (Ruan and Chen, 1998). Since most food systems are not in equilibrium, this frequently does not hold true.

Water mobility, as measured by nuclear magnetic resonance, is thought to be a more accurate way of determining the "availability" of water. Slade and Levine (1992) proposed the "polymer" approach to describe the role of water in food systems as a plasticizer that affects the glass transition temperature, which, in turn, could help explain the relationship between moisture and reaction rates (Nelson and Labuza, 1994).

In practice, the use of $a_w$ as a means to predict product stability remains important, while the polymer science approach can be viewed as a more generalized theoretical explanation (Reid, 1995). Water activity is a better indicator of food product susceptibility to spoilage than is water content. Dried foods normally contain 2 to 20 percent moisture, corresponding to $a_w$ in the range 0.20 to 0.60. In contrast, intermediate moisture foods (IMFs) normally contain 15 to 40 percent total moisture and have an $a_w$ of 0.60 to 0.85 (Jayaraman, 1995; Karel, 1973; Sloan et al., 1976).

## PROCESSING CONSIDERATIONS

Moisture control, mostly by dehydration, to lower the $a_w$ of the product is considered critical to attaining the required shelf life of the EFP of 2 to 3 years. The basic principle underlying drying and IMF technologies is the premise that water—the universal solvent—can become a limiting factor for spoilage and pathogenic microbial growth in foods when it is adequately reduced to low enough levels (Bone, 1973; Davies and Birch, 1976; Erickson, 1982; Gould, 1985; Rahman and Labuza, 1999). This reduction in moisture content and $a_w$ is sometimes accompanied by the use of other preservation factors such as chemical preservatives (e.g., antimicrobial agents, antioxidants, or antibrowning compounds), reduction of oxygen by vacuum and/or gas flushing techniques with maintenance through means of oxygen barrier packaging and/or oxygen-absorbent materials (oxygen scavengers), pH adjustment, and selection of packaging designs that protect the food from light, moisture, and environmental contamination. In the case of the EFP, moisture plays a critical role in determining microbial, sensory, chemical, and physical stability.

## Extrusion

High-temperature, short-time extrusion cooking has been extensively applied in IMF and dried food production. Basic phenomena in extrusion cooking have been described by many (Harper, 1978, 1979, 1988; Linko et al., 1981; Rossen and Miller, 1973; Smith, 1982). In an extruder, the raw food material is subjected simultaneously to heat, pressure, and shear within a short time. Desirable product functional characteristics are typically controlled by altering the feed composition and extrusion process parameters. Water is always an integral part of physicochemical processes (e.g., gelatinization of starch and protein denaturation and plasticization) that determine the final textural characteristics of an extruded product.

Extrusion can be applied to produce foods having various moisture levels, from dry IMF products (e.g., puffed snacks and ready-to-eat breakfast cereals) to soft, moist ones. Production of modern IMFs can belong to either one of three categories: (1) moist infusion, in which solid food pieces are soaked and/or cooked in a solution having low $a_w$, (2) dry infusion, where initial dehydration is followed by soaking the food in a solution having low $a_w$, and (3) blending, in which the components are weighed, blended, cooked, and extruded (Erickson, 1982). Extruded IMF products are also considered thermally processed as high-temperature, short-time (HTST). This not only helps to further preserve the product from potential microbial growth and adverse enzymatic action, but also can help reduce the amount of preservatives that would be necessary otherwise. HTST processes are rapid by definition, so little destruction of vitamins or loss of protein quality are expected. According to Harper (1988), heat-stable B vitamins and pantothenic acid are stable under extrusion conditions. However, oxidation of ascorbic acid or carotenoids could occur, particularly in puffed products, so puffed processing is not recommended for the EFP.

It may be possible to hot extrude some combination of the ingredients, such as a protein and carbohydrate mixture, and then combine it with other ingredients (e.g., fat) in a compressed bar. Microencapsulation might be used for some nutrients and flavors that are mixed into a compressed bar formulation, given that most encapsulation materials are not intended for heat-processed foods. Spray coating of some ingredients after heat processing might also provide ways of incorporating heat labile ingredients during manufacturing of the EFP, as is done in breakfast cereals (Caldwell et al., 2000). Thus, the more stable vitamins might be included in the extrusion mix and others incorporated later (e.g., ascorbic acid and thiamin).

## Maillard Browning Reaction

The Maillard reaction leads to brown color and to the appearance of new odors and flavors. The reaction involves reducing sugars and amino acids. It is a series of reactions that start with the formation of Amadori compounds from aldose or hexose carbonyl compounds condensing with free amino groups of amino acids or protein. The condensing product is a Schiffs base that later becomes aldosylamine, and this, in turn, is converted into ketosamines in the Amadori rearrangement. The final step involves formation of melanoidins, which are brown nitrogenous polymers or copolymers. Due to the complexity of Maillard reactions and their dependence on multiple factors (e.g., pH, temperature, composition of the medium, and moisture), it is difficult to predict the extent of browning. Sugars with different degrees of reducing power greatly influence the reaction kinetics. Water also affects it in a variety of ways. For example, a concentration of solids increases the reaction rate because of a reactant concentration effect; further concentration of solids leads to a reduced rate as the reactant mobility is decreased. In highly concentrated systems, the Maillard reaction is inhibited or retarded until, at some point, caramelization is more likely to occur than Maillard.

Generally, the activation energy of the Maillard reaction increases with decreasing moisture content, suggesting that mobility retardation may be the rate-limiting factor (Labuza and Saltmarch, 1981). There is an $a_w$ range where maximum Maillard reaction occurs that depends on: (a) the extent of the dilution effect at the high-moisture end, and (b) the limited mobility of reactants at the low-moisture end. For instance, the maximum $a_w$ range in apple is 0.53 to 0.55, whereas in dried anchovy it is 0.93 (Labuza, 1980). Unfortunately, most of the data available on reaction kinetics of the Maillard reaction is limited to $a_w$ values higher than 0.3 (Eichner and Karel, 1972; Warmbier et al., 1976). This suggests that if the EFP had an $a_w$ below 0.3, it would have an extended shelf life. Additionally, not much information is available on very high moisture systems that are believed to have slower reaction rates. From an equilibrium consideration, a Maillard reaction is not favored at high moisture because the advanced reaction and the early formation of a Schiff base involve removal of water (Hodge and Osman, 1976).

One of the nutritional implications of this reaction is a possible decreased digestibility and the loss of reactive amino acids, such as lysine (Kaanane and Labuza, 1989; Labuza 1994; Saltmarch and Labuza, 1982). This has been related to the cross linking of proteins, as demonstrated in freeze-dried meat (Barnett and Kim, 1997). In related work using an MRE chicken-a-la-king stored for 3 years between 4° and 30° C, Barnett and Kim (1997) reported that textural and sensory deterioration occurred much before the observed decrease in nutritive value. The $Q_{10}$ (i.e., the increase in the rate constant as temperature is increased by 10° C) in military MREs has been reported as 3 to 4, suggesting that under abusive storage conditions, a decrease in nutritive value in terms of reduced digestibility and loss of lysine can occur.

From the lysine-loss data, an estimation of the loss in nutritive value of the proteins in chicken meat heated at 73° C for 8 days in a high concentration of reducing sugar has been calculated to be about 13 percent (Barnett and Kim, 1997). If the above $Q_{10}$ is assumed for the browning reaction, heating for 8 days at 73° C would correspond to a storage for 22 years at an ambient temperature of 23° C, which exceeds the military shelf-life requirement of 3 years (ambient). Unfortunately, this information applies to chicken protein, but the EFP would contain only vegetable proteins. Therefore, the validity of this effect would need to be tested using EFP prototypes and conditions of storage and use simulating those expected during actual use of the EFP. Nevertheless, the key implication of this issue is that although the sensory quality may decrease and the nutritive value, to a lesser extent, may also be reduced because of the Maillard reaction, proper selection of ingredients for the EFP can help minimize sensory deterioration (e.g., appearance of brown color and firmer texture) and keep its nutritional quality from being adversely compromised.

## Microencapsulation

Microencapsulation provides a physical barrier to oxygen, metal catalysts, and other pro-oxidants. This type of technology has been used in the food industry for many years, but a wide range of patented processes have been developed in recent years (Brazel, 1999; Risch and Reineccius, 1995). The protection of nutrients and other unstable additives is made possible by microencapsulation formulations that can allow controlled release of the nutrient during digestion as well as preserve it during storage (Deasy, 1984; Kondo, 1979). By using microencapsulation, flavor, color, and texture can be improved, thus making the product more acceptable.

The selection of shell material for microencapsulated nutrients will depend on the material being protected, processing needs, and storage stability concerns (Brazel, 1999). Capsule shell-wall materials are food additives by definition, and include polysaccharides (e.g., alginates, agarose), proteins (e.g., caseinates, zein), and fats. The water or oil solubility of the component to be protected will dictate the shell material composition (Brazel, 1999).

Diffusion of oxygen and catalysts in the aqueous matrix of a food is dependent on the amorphous or crystalline nature of the aqueous phase (Shimada et al., 1991), and it has been proposed that the *glassy-rubbery* transition temperature ($T_g$—the temperature at which a rigid, amorphous, glassy material becomes molten and rubbery) plays a key role in governing oxidation of lipids embedded in the matrix (Roos and Karel, 1991). The free volume theory implies that gas diffusion through intermolecular spaces in the barrier (i.e., the continuous matrix in a dried micro-emulsion containing the oil droplets) depends on the glassy or rubbery state. As a glassy amorphous material undergoes a glass transition it gains a greater intermolecular freedom that can be described as the increase in molar free volume. A crystalline solid is a perfect barrier to diffusion and thus diffusion rate would depend on the intricacy of the barrier. In a system where water and oxygen diffusion occur simultaneously, the penetration front of water into a glassy, hydrophilic region would result in a decrease in $T_g$, with possible swelling or other structural change (e.g., collapse) at the hydration front as the polymer relaxes, transforming into a rubbery material depending on the time frame of the relaxation process with respect to diffusion time. This is expected to have a strong influence on oxygen diffusion (Chinachoti, 1998).

Therefore, migration of oxygen and other small molecules depends on polymer chain flexibility that can "flip-flop" according to local chain mobility, which creates openings or holes for small molecules to travel through. This mobility depends on the state of hydration.

The microstructure of microencapsulated oil has been reported to be a critical factor (Hardas et al., 2000, 2002; Ponginebbi et al., 2000). Oxidation rates of surface and encapsulated lipids have been shown to follow various mechanisms depending on the physical integrity and mobility of the matrix. Hence, the effect of moisture on oxidation of surface and encapsulated lipid fractions can vary widely (Hardas et al., 2002).

Vitamins and minerals are often encapsulated to prevent unpleasant flavors and to prevent oxidation. Labile components such as fat-soluble vitamins are blended with lipids in emulsion droplets as part of the encapsulation process. Proper selection of surfactants that are antioxidants is advised, and care must be taken to ensure emulsion stability. To prevent easy moisture penetration, the encapsulation matrices should not have a low $T_g$. However, for enhanced bioavailability, they should disintegrate upon rehydration in the mouth or upon adding water. Capsule materials that ensure release of the nutrient during digestion are usually hydrophobic fats or waxes, but some cellulose and protein derivatives can be used (Brazel, 1999).

Microencapsulation has been shown to greatly retard the oxidation of some oils that are rich in unsaturated and polyunsaturated fatty acids (Lin et al., 1995; Velasco et al., 2000). Typically, the oil is homogenized in water with the aid of an emulsifier and the resultant mixture is rapidly dried—most often in a spray drier—to yield a powdered, encapsulated product. Numerous encapsulation formulas have been tried; those that result in the highest amount of oil in the core of the particle have the best stability. Combination of antioxidants such as Δ-tocopherol (Han et al., 1991) and ascorbic acid or α-tocopherol and ascorbyl palmitate (Kaitaranta, 1992) may be used for additional protection. However, very few investigations have focused on the effect of storage and antioxidants on the oxidation of surface (free) and encapsulated lipids in microencapsulated fish oil (Velasco et al., 2000). In addition, the physical changes from amorphous to crystalline discussed above are factors that remain to be further investigated in order to improve product stability.

Coating or encapsulation is routinely done in the manufacture of fortification nutrients and flavors, but because the techniques are proprietary, it is difficult to find specific studies in the scientific literature. The primary reasons for encapsulation are to prevent interactions with other nutrients, prevent losses due to oxidation or moisture, and to minimize undesirable flavors from vitamins or minerals. The type of coating or capsule used is dependent on the compound, and to a lesser extent, the matrix (Meyers, 1998). Vitamin C (ascorbic acid) is most often coated with fat or Ethocel to provide stability against oxidation. Vitamin K encapsulated in gum acacia is available on the market.

### Stable Nutrient Forms

Stable nutrient forms, other than encapsulated, may also include metal chelates such as sodium iron EDTA (NaFe EDTA), which has been shown to be effective in reducing anemia, particularly in diets high in phytates, without adversely affecting other minerals (Davidsson et al., 1994, 1998; Hurrell et al., 2000). Iron chelates have been tested in various feeding situations and found to enhance absorption of soluble iron fortificants, such as ferrous sulfate or ferrous fumarate. For example, both NaFeEDTA and $Na_2EDTA$ were effective enhancers of iron absorption from cereal foods (Davidsson et al., 2001a, 2001b; Hurrell et al., 2000). Ascorbic acid had a similar effect in high-phytate foods (Davidsson et al., 2001a, 2001b; Hurrell et al., 2000).

## MICROBIOLOGICAL CONSIDERATIONS

The addition of small amounts of solutes and dehydration are two main methods of decreasing $a_w$ and of increasing osmotic pressure in a food system to inhibit microbial growth. Reduced availability of water contributes to impaired microbial growth, and hence it has been used widely as a microbiological safety parameter (Beuchat, 1987; Gould, 1985; Lenovich, 1987; Troller, 1987; Troller and Christian, 1978). However, $a_w$ is not a universal parameter but rather an empirical one (Franks, 1982). The efficacy of manipulating $a_w$ is limited to certain types of microorganisms and is affected by food composition and environmental conditions (Andrews and Pitt, 1987; Corry, 1978; Vaamonde et al., 1982), and by the presence of microbial inhibitors (Leistner, 1995). Hence, there is no single minimum $a_w$ for inhibiting microbial growth that can be applied to all foods and all microorganisms.

It is generally accepted that bacteria are more susceptible to osmotic effects than are molds and yeasts (with some exceptions). For IMF products, the main pathogenic bacterium of concern is *Staphylococcus aureus*, which can produce serious food poisoning if a significant amount of its enterotoxin is ingested. *S. aureus*, implicated in 20 to 40 percent of all foodborne illness outbreaks in the United States (Lavoie et al., 1997), is able to grow at an $a_w$ as low as 0.85. Additionally, yeasts and molds, particularly the xerophilic kind (those that prefer dry ambient conditions), survive and grow in moisture-limited environments. The lowest $a_w$ values at which mold growth may occur, albeit very slowly, are 0.61 to 0.62 (Pitt and Christian, 1968), whereas mold sporulation does not take place at $a_w$ less than 0.75 (Pitt, 1975).

In addition to $a_w$, factors influencing microbial survival and growth have been investigated with respect to water mobility, the translational or rotational motion of water molecules (Lavoie et al., 1997; Pham et al., 1999). It has been demonstrated that water mobility may influence transport of nutrients to microbial cells and hence growth. Under conditions of limited moisture, mold spore germination and mycelial growth strongly correlate with water mobility (Pham et al., 1999). For the EFP, the type and composition of ingredients used will influence the interaction of solids with water, thereby affecting water mobility and $a_w$, and thus the survival and potential growth of pathogenic microorganisms. More importantly, should spores or vegetative cells of microorganisms able to withstand dry conditions survive the processing, they could germinate and grow during storage if moisture is not properly controlled in the product and other provisions, such as addition of preservatives, are not made to inhibit microbial growth. To minimize the risk of biological hazards, a multiple hurdle approach is highly recommended (Leistner, 1995). In this approach, also called the combined methods approach, several factors are used together to inhibit microbial growth, such as thermal processing, plus $a_w$, storage temperature, preservatives, and packaging. For the EFP, it can be expected that there will be little, if any, opportunity to control storage temperature and ambient humidity. On the other hand, the cost of production and materials (including packaging) that would be incurred in making an IMF-type EFP might be too high, and there would also be a price to pay in terms of product shelf life and safety. As pointed out earlier, dehydration and IMF technologies can only stop microorganisms from growing but do not necessarily inactivate them. Consequently, and although an EFP having IMF characteristics should not be ruled out as an option, ***the optimal approach to the microbiological stability of the EFP would be a product design having an $a_w$ value lower than those in the IMF range (e.g., 0.4) and to add some preservatives***.

## CHEMICAL STABILITY CONSIDERATIONS

### Lipid Oxidation

Auto-oxidation of lipids occurs in foods largely via a self-propagating free radical mechanism. Since direct reaction of unsaturated linkages in lipids with oxygen is energetically difficult, production of the first few radicals needed to start the propagation reaction must occur through some catalytic mechanism (Nawar, 1996). It has been proposed that the initiation step may take place by decomposition to free radicals of preformed hydroperoxides via metal catalysis or heat, by exposure to light, by direct reaction of metals with oxidizable substrates, or by mechanisms where singlet oxygen is the active species involved (Nawar, 1996).

Upon formation of sufficient free radicals, a chain reaction is initiated by the abstraction of hydrogen atoms at positions alpha to double bonds followed by oxygen attack at these locations. The result is production of peroxy radicals,

ROO•, which in turn abstract hydrogen from α-methylenic groups or other molecules, RH, to form hydroperoxides, ROOH, and yield R• groups that react with oxygen, and so on. Due to resonance stabilization of the R• species, the reaction is usually accompanied by shifting in the position of double bonds resulting in the formation of isomeric hydroperoxides that often contain conjugated diene groups.

Lipid oxidation gives rise to formation of a number of breakdown products, some of which are responsible for various off-flavors known as rancidity (Nawar, 1996). Even if only a single type of substrate is involved (e.g., one unsaturated fatty acid), the rate and pathway of its oxidation will depend on many factors that include its molecular structure (i.e., the number and location of double bonds), concentration, type of oxidant, oxygen tension, temperature, surface area, pH, time, physical state, and pro- and antioxidants present (Nawar, 1996).

Numerous antioxidant compounds have been studied, including α-tocopherol, α-tocopherol acetate, ascorbyl palmitate, butylated hydroxytoluene, butylated hydroxyanisole, di-t-butylhydroquinone, green tea catechins, and flavonoids, with mixed results (Lindsay, 1996). Briefly, it appears that the degree of oxidation inhibition apparently attained with antioxidants is affected by the method used to measure it and on the system studied.

## Effect of Moisture on Lipid Oxidation

Although moisture reduction may discourage or inhibit microorganisms from growing in a food during storage, the moisture that remains may promote some chemical reactions such as nonenzymatic browning and enzymatic reactions. Depending on the system, these reactions are normally slowed down at low $a_w$ values, and, in general, at $a_w$ < BET[1], the rates can be very slow and the product may remain in good condition through extended storage if it is properly formulated, processed, and packaged.

There is one exception, however, with respect to oxidative deterioration of lipids and fat-soluble nutrients. It has been shown that lipid oxidation can be increasingly high at moisture levels below a "critical $a_w$" (Nelson and Labuza, 1992a, 1992b). This critical $a_w$ value is reached when a reduction in the moisture content is accompanied by a decrease in the oxidation rate up to a minimum. At moisture levels below this point, oxidation may rise again. Thus, there is a line of demarcation for lowering $a_w$: in the $a_w$ range of 0.2 to 0.3, lipid oxidation is likely to be accelerated, whereas at $a_w$ between 0.3 and 0.6, lipid oxidation and other deteriorative reactions are minimized. There are a number of proposed explanations for this effect that implicate the state of hydration of catalysts (e.g.,

---

[1] Brunauer-Emmett-Teller value, normally 4 to 5 percent moisture (Brunauer et al., 1938).

metals) and hydroperoxides, phase transition, mobilization of pro- and antioxidants, and diffusion-related phenomena (Fritsch, 1994).

In the case of the EFP, oxidative changes in the lipid phase would be of concern when unsaturated lipids and minerals are present in significant amounts, for not only could they lead to adverse changes in flavor and acceptability, but also to production of toxic by-products and destruction of fat-soluble vitamins (Gregory, 1996). Therefore, although products at an intermediate moisture range may be more appealing in sensory quality, they may also be more prone to spoilage, browning, and other reactions. On the other hand, lowering the water content of the product to a dry state (< 5 percent moisture) may promote lipid oxidation. A solution to this dilemma would be to develop a dry product (< 5 percent moisture) in which lipids and pro-oxidants are kept separate by means of physical barriers, such as in encapsulation. Use of antioxidants also may be necessary depending on the level of saturation of the lipids. Additionally, the packaging method and materials used would play an important role in the oxidative stability of the EFP (Burke, 1990). The advantages of a dry product must be weighed against the fact that, for a thirsty recipient, eating it may be an unpleasant experience.

It should be noted that in the event the product is amenable to hydration before consumption, its microbiological safety should be evaluated. Potential growth of pathogenic microorganisms after rehydration—particularly if the product is not immediately consumed—could pose serious health risks, especially for recipients having impaired immune systems and vulnerable subgroups such as young children and the elderly.

***Because of the above considerations, it is advisable that the lipids and pro-oxidants (e.g,. added mineral ingredients) in the EFP be kept physically separated within the product during manufacturing and subsequent storage by encapsulation of the minerals***. Careful design of the encapsulation materials will be required so that they cover the intended ingredients efficiently, hold their integrity under the selected processing conditions, and disintegrate upon consumption so that nutrients are made physiologically available. Further protection against oxidation of unsaturated fats and vitamins in the EFP may be accomplished through a combination of microencapsulation, use of suitable antioxidants, development of stable emulsion prior to drying, and appropriate packaging.

## Nutrient Stability During Processing and Storage

Experimental data on vitamin stability and degradation kinetics have been extensively reviewed (Karmas and Harris, 1988; Kirk, 1981; Villota and Hawkes, 1992). The nutritional quality of dehydrated foods is a function of temperature, light, oxygen, moisture, and the physicochemical state of the water (Bluestein and Labuza, 1988). The various chemical forms of added nutrients are subjected to degradation differently (Gregory, 1996). The description below reflects some major aspects of the degradation kinetics of nutrients related to the effect of moisture.

Experiments have been conducted on the effects of long-term storage at 4.4°, 21.1°, and 37.8° C, nutritional quality, oxidative and browning reactions, and sensory quality of fruit cake and chocolate brownies (Salunkhe et al., 1979). When stored in retort pouches at 37.8° C , the approximate half-life for thiamin was 30 months (fruit cake) or 15 months (chocolate brownies); for riboflavin and niacin, the half-life was less than 30 months in both products. However, the products were unacceptable due to off-flavor, dryness, and rancidity at about the half-life time for thiamin (at this point, rancidity had doubled). This indicates that the shelf life of this type of product could be less than 6 months when stored in a hot environment (e.g., 37° C), and that additional deterrents such as dehydration, reduction of $a_w$, and others might be necessary to provide vitamin stability.

Fat-soluble vitamins, particularly vitamins A and E, exhibit stability similar to unsaturated fat. Their degradation rates significantly increase with increasing $a_w$ values from very low (~0) to 0.4. Temperature can also greatly influence their destruction; their activation energy is in the range 10 to 25 kcal/mol and decreases with increasing $a_w$. In the presence of metal catalysts, the degradation kinetics of vitamin A are not affected if the $a_w$ is kept adequately low so that the catalyst is immobilized (Kirk, 1981; Labuza, 1971).

In the case of water-soluble vitamins, their degradation is dependent on the state of the water (free to act as a solvent for reactants and catalysts or bound) and the $a_w$ in the system. Degradation of thiamin seems to be enhanced when a Maillard-type browning is observed, which is to say, when reactants are mobile. A study by Kirk (1981) indicated that when thiamin, vitamin A, and riboflavin are used in fortification of dehydrated foods, very little degradation (< 2 percent loss) takes place at an $a_w$ in the range 0.1 to 0.4 and storage in paperboard boxes at 30° C. However, at a higher temperature (37° C), a significant decrease in vitamin retention was observed with an increasing $a_w$ over the same range. Ascorbic acid degradation studies in a dry model food system indicated that the rate of degradation of this nutrient increased with increasing relative humidity of storage or increasing initial moisture content (Purwadaria et al., 1979).

Therefore, based on the information available, some conclusions may be advanced regarding retention of nutrients that will need to be confirmed when the exact prototypes of the EFP are developed. ***First, to ensure nutrient retention, $a_w$ may need to be kept lower than 0.4; the lower the $a_w$, the more stable some of the nutrients would be***. This is more critical in tropical and arid areas, where storage of the EFP at elevated temperatures could accelerate the degradation process. In addition, this low $a_w$ would be in agreement with that necessary to provide protection against microbial growth in the EFP. ***A higher $a_w$ (e.g., up to 0.6) may be used if there are compelling reasons to do so and its***

***influence on stability and shelf life of the EFP are determined***. Second, it might be possible to apply microencapsulation technology to add additional oxygen barriers to labile components such as fat-soluble vitamins, always keeping a low $a_w$ (< 0.4) in the product. Third, for water-soluble vitamins, it is most critical that water mobility be kept low again by keeping $a_w$ adequately low (< 0.4), and that minerals are encapsulated. Minerals are unlikely to be influenced by $a_w$, since they are stable during most processing and storage regimens.

***Testing of EFPs must be conducted throughout the expected shelf life of the EFP and under conditions of delivery and storage simulating actual use, to ascertain the initial content and stability of nutrients***. Standard methodologies for determining vitamin and mineral content are well described in the literature, and appropriate procedures, such as those used for nutritional labeling, can be applied to the EFP. Determining bioavailability of micronutrients from the EFP is not a feasible outcome of its development and manufacture, given the complex issue of such testing (Van Campen and Glahn, 1999).

## ACCEPTABILITY CONSIDERATIONS

The characteristics of a food product (i.e., appearance, flavor, and texture), the conditions under which it is consumed, and the appeal that it has for a specific consumer determine its acceptance. Measurement of liking, described below, is used during product development to predict consumer response before investments are made in equipment, production, and distribution (Stone and Sidel, 1993).

### Measurement of Liking

Preference and liking are generally thought to be almost the same, and techniques used for their measurement are often similar (Peryam, 1998). However, preference implies a choice between products, without considering how well liked each one is. Therefore, measurement of the degree of liking, or "hedonic value," is a means of determining not only whether one food is preferred to another, but how acceptable or well liked it is.

In the 1950s, considerable work was done at the U.S. Army Quartermaster Food and Container Institute to establish methodology for predicting soldiers' food choices (Peryam and Girardot, 1952). The relevance and reliability of the hedonic scale method, based on known rating scale methods used in psychology, were established through extensive field testing of army rations of all types (Peryam and Pilgrim, 1957). Since the development of the technique, the nine-point hedonic scale has been used extensively and validated by numerous studies of food products. Although there are still issues regarding its use, it remains one of the most useful tools for determining consumer acceptance (Lawless and Heymann, 1999; Meilgaard et al., 1999; Stone and Sidel, 1993).

In hedonic rating, testers are presented with a continuous or discrete scale with nine marked points, where 1 is "dislike extremely," 5 is "neither like or dislike," and 9 is "like extremely" (Peryam and Pilgrim, 1957). Other points are like or dislike "very much," "moderately," or "slightly." Testers are asked to respond to the food product on this scale and express their honest opinion of liking. They are reassured that there is no correct answer. The data are then interpreted numerically and analyzed statistically.

Interpretation of hedonic testing results is open to debate. At what value on the nine-point scale does a product become unacceptable, and when is it an excellent product? According to Peryam (Peryam and Girardot, 1952; Peryam and Pilgrim, 1957), a hedonic rating less than 4.5 is unacceptable, while an ordinary staple food would range between 6.25 and 7.25. Interpretation is based on the food product; some items, such as candy and ice cream, would be expected to achieve averages higher than 7.25 or be poor prospects.

Prediction of food consumption is an area of continuing research in both food and behavioral sciences. Cardello and colleagues (2000) pointed out that food preference and acceptability testing may not be a successful indication of consumer behavior towards consumption. However, affective tests of liking remain an integral part of food product development and marketing. Cardello and coworkers (2000) found that predicting consumer behavior toward foods in real-life situations is difficult and that standard methods of determining liking in controlled situations may not be reliable. In the case of the EFP, it will not be possible to test the product in a real-life situation. However, ***testing under conditions similar to those used by the U.S. Army for GP Survival Packets and MREs is recommended***.

## Shelf-Life Testing

The length of time that a product is acceptable and meets consumer expectations of its quality is considered to be its shelf life (Labuza, 1982). Procedures for determining shelf life comprise microbiological, chemical, and sensory testing to give an objective point for stating that the product does not meet expected quality. In general, microbiological and sensory endpoints are used. Criteria for determining shelf life must be determined prior to starting the process. However, moisture content, $a_w$, lipid oxidation, and vitamin losses can be correlated with sensory changes and serve as indices of stability (Giese, 2000).

A standard guide for shelf-life determination by sensory methods is being considered by the ASTM E-18 Committee (1997), which describes criteria and experimental design considerations for real-time and accelerated shelf-life testing. For products expected to have an extended storage time, such as the

EFP, accelerated testing is needed (Labuza and Schmidl, 1985). The concept behind these tests is that subjecting foods to a controlled environment in which temperature or humidity, for example, is higher than normal causes an increased deterioration rate. At least one characteristic (e.g., sensory quality, vitamin content, or oxidative rancidity) must be measured analytically so that a prediction model can be built (Labuza and Schmidl, 1988; Ragnarsson and Labuza, 1977). Based on the accelerated testing, a prediction of the storage stability of the product can be made. Other models are available: Nelson and Labuza (1994) examined two models for determining the effects of $a_w$ on shelf life, while others (Cardelli and Labuza, 2001; Duyvestyen et al., 2001; Gacula, 1975a, 1975b; Gacula and Singh, 1984) have evaluated the Weibull Hazard Analysis proposed for use in shelf-life testing by Gacula in 1975.

***The critical issue for the EFP is maintenance of eating and nutritional quality. Shelf-life testing for the product, therefore, should be based on both of these criteria, as well as on microbiological safety for an at-risk population.*** The suggestion made by the U.S. Army to use its facilities at various overseas locations to test the EFP among local populations, so that its acceptability by populations having diverse ethnic and cultural backgrounds can be evaluated, seems to be a realistic method to evaluate the prototypes.

## PACKAGING CONSIDERATIONS

### EFP Configuration and Packaging

The EFP will be used in environments that exhibit a wide range of temperature and humidity conditions, including extreme environments, often characterized by a lack of a delivery infrastructure. Therefore, all packaging components must be capable of withstanding a wide range of temperatures (Riordan, 1970) and physical abuse. In addition, these food items will be delivered by various modes of transportation, including airdrop. Separate packaging, or more likely, additional packaging, may be necessary for EFP airdrop operations.

The first step in defining packaging requirements is to define a product configuration for product delivery and the use and protection requirements for each component. The starting point in the configuration for the EFP is a daily ration required to provide 2,100 kcal along with proteins, lipids, vitamins, and minerals to maintain nutritional status. This unit must be protected for a 3-year shelf life, and because of the product's dual susceptibility to moisture and oxygen, moisture and oxygen must be removed from the product environment before or during packaging and essentially excluded throughout its storage life. The ration is likely to be a low-moisture product (< 5 percent) that achieves microbiological stability through limited $a_w$ (< 0.4), and includes polyunsaturated fatty acids, which are prone to oxidation. Moisture should be restricted through the initial formulation. Oxygen, on the other hand, must be removed during the packaging operation by drawing a vacuum, flushing with nitrogen, or both. A high barrier to both moisture and oxygen transmission is also essential to protect the product post-packaging.

Oxidation of food components is curtailed in low-oxygen environments, as described earlier. Oxygen levels below 1 percent have been found to reduce oxidation sufficiently to provide stability for unsaturated fatty acids (Brody, 1989). Some molds can grow at oxygen levels as low as 0.1 percent and produce mycotoxins (Nielsen et al., 1989). Oxygen levels of 0.2 to 0.5 percent (2,000 to 5,000 ppm) can be achieved using vacuum and vacuum plus gas flush technologies for solid products. Initial oxygen concentrations at these levels can be obtained for porous products as well, but degassing of these products (i.e., gas losses by the product itself) may quickly raise the initial oxygen concentrations into the 1 to 2 percent range. Salame (1974) suggested that dried foods required protection to restrict oxygen gain to a maximum of 5 to 15 ppm and could tolerate a maximum moisture gain of 1 percent over their shelf life.

Acceptably low oxygen levels can be maintained only with packaging materials having sufficient barrier properties. The initial oxygen level and the upper limit of oxygen to be permitted in the package must be set in specifying actual barrier requirements. The necessary oxygen barrier to limit oxygen influx to 10 ppm over 3 years for the EFP would require an essentially perfect barrier to oxygen. More realistically, ***to maintain an oxygen level below 2 percent for the expected 3-year shelf life of the EFP at 23° C (70° F) in a 10×10×5-cm configuration, which yields 500 cc (450 cc for a product having an approximate density of 1.0 and a 50-cc allowance for primary wraps), and assuming a pouch surface area of 400 cm$^2$, for example, and an initial oxygen concentration of 0.1 percent, sufficient barrier is achieved with a maximum oxygen transmission of 0.00088 cc/100 in$^2$/day***.

Such a barrier can be achieved using glass, metal, or thick films of high-barrier polymers. Glass packaging would be inappropriate for the EFP because of excessive weight, field disposal, and fragility. Rigid metal or plastic containers are contraindicated for similar reasons. This leaves flexible materials: aluminum foil, high-barrier polymers, and metalized films. ***The optimal choice for barrier and cost reasons is an aluminum foil laminate*** (Lampi, 1977; Szczeblowski, 1971).

To be sufficiently thick, high-barrier polymers such as ethylene vinyl alcohol or polyvinylidene chloride would be too costly and too bulky. "Metalized" films, in turn, can be prepared with excellent barrier properties if—and only if—the metalization completely covers the substrate. Typically, these films would be able to provide moderate, but not sufficient, barrier for use in the EFP. Therefore, aluminum foil would be the choice material.

Aluminum foils range in thickness from 4.3 μm (0.00017 in) to 150 μm (0.0059 in). By industry definition, rolled aluminum becomes foil at a thickness below 152.4 μm (0.006 in). Foils exhibit pinholes as a function of thickness.

When foils are rolled to gauges below 10 µm, the incidence of pinholes increases exponentially (Anderson, 1988). Studies conducted in 1961 and 1985 showed that improvements in rolling techniques reduced the incidence of pinholes for thin foils (Anderson, 1988). For example, approximately 200 pinholes were observed per square meter with 9-µm foils in 1961, whereas a similar performance was obtained with 8-µm foils in 1985.

Foils are considered impermeable at a thickness of 25.4 µm (0.001 in) and above. At 8.9 µm (0.00035 in), the water vapor transmission rate (WVTR) is equal to or below 0.065 cc/m$^2$ (0.02 cc/100 in$^2$)/day at 37.8° C (100° F) (Brody and Marsh, 1997). These values drop if foil is laminated to appropriate polymeric materials. ***The thickness for the foil layer, therefore, could be within the range 8.8 to 18.0 µm (0.00035 to 0.0007 in), which provides the needed barrier at the lowest thickness, and therefore, at the lowest cost.*** Within this thickness range, foils still exhibit minor pinholes (Anderson, 1988), but lamination with polyolefin provides sufficient protection from influx of oxygen. At a thickness of 0.00035 in, aluminum foil was reported to present pinholes of approximately 0.00004 in$^2$/100 in$^2$. Marsh (1996) calculated that a 1-mil polypropylene coating applied to a foil substrate with an effective surface area for permeation of 0.00004 in$^2$/100 in$^2$ of film would exhibit reduced transmission values of 0.0076 cc/100 in$^2$/day/atm for oxygen and 0.00002 cc/100 in$^2$/day/atm for water vapor. These transmission rates are expected to be sufficient to maintain an oxygen level below 2 percent and to provide acceptable protection against moisture influx for 3 years at 23° C.

Aluminum foil is fragile and prone to tearing unless it is protected. A tough polymer—toughness being defined as the area under the stress strain curve (Marin and Sauer, 1954)—can provide both puncture and tear protection to aluminum foil. Two applicable polymers are polyethylene terephthalate (polyester) and polyamides (nylon). According to Lampi (1977), a 0.0005-in thick film laminated to the outside of the foil via extrusion or adhesives would provide sufficient protection: an $O_2$ transmission rate below 1 cc/100 in$^2$/atm/day (15.5 cc/m$^2$/day) and a WVTR below 0.05 cc/100 in$^2$/day. Compared to the numbers given in the paragraph above, and by current standards, these specifications for barrier properties appear to be high. However, the apparent discrepancy is easily resolved after considering that Lampi's values represented an untested level. The verification of low water and oxygen transmission was through sensory testing rather than permeation testing (Szczeblowski, 1971). Additionally, the limit of permeation detectability in the 1970s was lower than today. In 1970, the level of oxygen transmission detectability was 0.003 cc/100 in$^2$/day (0.0456 cc/m$^2$/day); in 2001 the level of detectability was 0.00003 cc/100 in$^2$/day (0.0005 cc/m$^2$/day) (personal communication, MOCON, 2001). Foil laminates, therefore, would have measured below the limits of detectability in the earlier work.

As a result of the above discussion, ***a trilaminate structure that has been extensively tested for long shelf-life food applications is recommended for the EFP*** (Lampi, 1977; Szczeblowski, 1971). Because lamination costs are related to quantity, primarily because short-run set-up charges can render lamination costs prohibitive, the trilaminate currently used by the military is recommended (from inside to outside: 0.003- to 0.004-in thick polyolefin/0.00035- to 0.00078-in thick aluminum foil/0.0005-in thick polyester [Natick Research, Development, and Engineering Center, 1993]). Other laminations with the recommended properties are also applicable, including the enhanced laminate currently recommended by the military that uses both polyester and nylon for additional protection against distribution (mechanical) forces. ***The package should be nitrogen flushed, and residual oxygen must not exceed 0.5 percent.***

***A notch in the package seal must be provided to facilitate opening by EFP recipients, who would likely have no scissors or other tools at their disposal.***

## Individual EFP Bars

Although the EFP has been designed to provide 2,100 kcal/day to recipients as a daily ration of approximately 450 g, it should be divided into smaller units for a number of reasons. First, considering that most people would normally eat more than one meal during the course of the day, dividing the daily ration into smaller portions provides for multiple meals. Second, it facilitates feeding children who need smaller amounts to meet energy needs. Third, it helps prevent the entire ration from being exposed when only part of it is going to be consumed. Therefore, ***it is suggested that the ration be divided into equal portions having the shape of bars***. To facilitate packaging, ***nine bars would be appropriate***. To further facilitate division of portions for young children, ***each individual bar should be centrally scored across the width of the bar to provide two 116-cal portions upon breaking it.***

***Each one of the nine bars should be wrapped in a primary packaging***—defined as the package that is in intimate contact with the product (Saroka, 1999)—that does not need to be a barrier material. (Lampi [1977] defined the pouch and carton used for retort pouches as the "immediate container" in the EFP application, the immediate container would include this primary wrap, the barrier container for each daily ration, and the bundling bag for multiple days or people.) It is recommended that this primary wrap be pulp-based and have a moisture-barrier coating. Individual bars could be wrapped in polyethylene or wax-coated paper (Fennema and Kester, 1991) as an unsealed wrapping similar to the inner wrapping of a candy bar. This wrap would provide a minor moisture barrier for individual bars after the EFP trilaminate is opened. More importantly, it would separate individual bars for easier access and would prevent microbial contamination from insects, handling, and surroundings. In addition to separating individual bars, the wrappings could be used by refugees or victims of emergencies to start fires for cooking or providing heat.

The secondary packaging is defined as that which bundles the primary packages (Saroka, 1999). ***A daily supply of nine bars should be packaged together under a nitrogen flush or vacuum into a barrier package*** to provide the barrier against oxygen and moisture needed for extended shelf life. The secondary packaging could be a pouch having a similar construction to that of the trilaminate pouch utilized by the military for long shelf-life rations, which consists, from the inside out, of polyolefin, aluminum foil, and polyester or nylon (defined above). This daily supply is considered a "unit."

## Five-Day EFP Package for Distribution

Anecdotal evidence provided by relief agencies indicates the convenience of grouping five daily rations into a single bundle. The rationale for this selection is that it permits 5 days worth of food for a single individual or 1 day of feeding a five-member family to be distributed as a unit. In addition, it is desirable to have a distribution-bundled package that is not easily carried by soldiers or personnel for which the EFP is not intended. Therefore, it is recommended that ***five EFP daily rations be bundled into a monoaxially- or biaxially-oriented polyolefin bag. The bag should be notched to facilitate opening***.

A rigid container could be used for the bundling instead of the polymeric bag. This could be a rigid plastic or metal container. Although such containers would add weight, they offer additional protection against rodents and may also serve additional purposes after consumption of the EFPs, such as carrying water. This option becomes especially attractive if such use (e.g., as a water carrier) replaces or precludes a separate delivery of such items.

## Shipping Containers

***Eight bundles of five EFPs each will be placed into a shipping container to constitute a case. The shippers could be of corrugated construction, sufficient to pass distribution protocols of ASTM International or the International Safe Transit Association***. Their dimensions will depend upon the actual shape of the bars, which is not specified in this performance-based recommendation. It is anticipated that single-wall, C-flute corrugate would suffice. Each shipper will weigh in the vicinity of 40 lb. Shipping containers could also be constructed of metal so that they can be recycled for use as storage or water containers as suggested by anecdotal evidence.

## Pallets

Shippers will be assembled onto a pallet for transport. ***Pallets will be of construction and dimensions to provide efficient transport, with overhang and underhang restricted to a maximum of 2 in***. Approximately 50 cases will be placed on a pallet. Pallets may be unitized using stretch wrap, banding, adhesive, or other means.

## Airdrop

### Naked Rations

Depending upon the ultimate shape and density of the EFP, it should be possible to airdrop individual EFP packs in ways similar to MREs, using the Triad (tri-wall aerial distribution system) that was used to airdrop food in Bosnia (Roos, 1993). Individual MREs were found to fall with a terminal velocity of 58 mph, which was suitable for delivery. The tri-wall distribution container was used to transport the MREs, but was not included in the drop. This method may be applicable if the terminal velocity of the EFP is found to be sufficiently low to allow for safe delivery. However, given the caloric density requirements of the EFP, it is anticipated that it will be a heavy product such that additional packaging protection will be required for air delivery in this manner.

### Flutter Packs

The World Food Programme developed a plastic film tube package with unequal amounts of food product sealed into each end. The length of tube between the product catches air during free fall and slows the descent. The unequal product weights cause a precessing (whirling) motion that absorbs energy during the free fall, thus the package name. However, because the weight of product delivered using this system is less than that of the EFP, its applicability for EFP delivery must be tested.

### Wing Packs

Alternate configurations to the Flutter Pack may be developed that provide sufficient wind resistance to slow descent to a safe level.

### Bubble Packs

Bubble packs or suitable cushioning material may be layered such that impact is attenuated as successive layers absorb impact and rupture. This would constitute an individual pack adaptation of the airbag approach that has been developed for bulk delivery (see below). Dimensions of bubbles, pressure of enclosed gas (which would change with altitude), and strength of substrate that will rupture must all be determined to prove efficacy for specific ration configurations (single or multiple) and specified drop heights. Drop height may be extended if terminal velocity is acceptable.

### Cushion Packs

Additional cushioning materials may be employed to attenuate impact to acceptable levels for EFP delivery. These cushions could be composed of a variety of materials (thermoset or thermoplastic foams, rubber, cellulosic), composites, or constructions (such as paperboard honeycomb, mentioned below). Two considerations are required for suitability, however: the integrity of the EFP and the safety of the delivery. Unless remote delivery is assured, the airdrop must not present a hazard to the intended recipients.

## Bulk Drops

### Cushion

The steady descent velocity experienced with parachute airdrops is about 28 ft/sec (Lee, 1992). Ground impact at this velocity requires an energy absorber to dissipate the impact energy. An evaluation of cushioning materials by Ellis and coworkers (1961) concluded that paperboard honeycomb was the most cost-effective, all-around, airdrop, energy-dissipating material. A majority of U.S. Army airdrops are delivered by the Container Delivery System, which has a 2,000-lb payload and uses honeycomb protection. Other cushioning materials may also prove adequate, but ***any material will require evaluation to assure proper loading and effectiveness under the environmental conditions that may be expected during the airdrops***.

### Foam

The U.S. Army evaluated alternatives to cushions because of specific shortcomings. Cushioning materials take up substantial warehouse space, are labor-intensive to use (primarily for equipment loads that require assembly, but would be less of a concern with uniform loads for items such as the EFP), and may degrade in high humidity (especially the paperboard honeycomb). Foams offers an alternative that overcomes these difficulties (Goldberg, 1990). As mentioned above, testing would be necessary to determine loading and use conditions.

### Air Bag

Another option for airdrop impact reduction is air bags. This option utilizes the restricted venting of the air bag to reduce impact forces. Complex air bags using vent control and/or gas injection, and augmented air bags using paperboard honeycomb or other cushioning, have been found to improve the performance of simple air bags by decreasing peak gravity forces (Lee, 1992). Such systems offer further alternatives for bulk air drops of the EFP that could be evaluated when prototypes are prepared.

## COST CONSIDERATIONS

The goal of this report is to develop an EFP that has an optimal nutritional profile and could meet the most severe environmental, storage, and logistic conditions. However, it is recognized that the requirements to produce such a sophisticated product are substantial. If funds are limited, a high unit cost can dramatically reduce the quantity of rations available to a needy population. Given this concern, the technical specifications recommended in this report should be considered optimal; however, the sponsoring agencies may choose to consider developing EFPs prepared and packaged to less stringent specifications if cost becomes a primary consideration. Under these circumstances, an EFP packaged in airtight foil bags inside a water-repellent paperboard box, for example, would allow greater quantities of products to be procured for a fixed cost and would be adequate in many relief situations, particularly for disaster relief. However, in this case, the long shelf-life objective and possibly also the goal of prepositioning supplies around the world would have to be modified by the agencies.

## REFERENCES


Anderson AN. 1988. Typical causes of pinholes in pack rolled foil©. *Lubr Eng* 44:622–625.

Andrews S, Pitt JI. 1987. Further studies on the water relationships of xerophilic fungi, including some halophiles. *J Gen Microbiol* 133:233–238.

ASTM E-18 Committee. 1997. *Proposed Standard Guide for Shelf Life Determination*. Philadelphia: ASTM.

Barnett RE, Kim H-J. 1997. Protein instability. In: Taub IA, Singh RP, eds. *Food Storage Stability*. Boca Raton, FL: CRC Press. Pp. 75–87.

Beuchat LR. 1987. Influence of water activity on sporulation, germination, outgrowth, and toxin production. In: Rockland LB, Beuchat LR, eds. *Water Activity: Theory and Applications to Food*. New York: Marcel Dekker. Pp. 137–151.

Bluestein PM, Labuza TP. 1988. Effects of moisture removal on nutrients. In: Karmas E, Harris RS, eds. *Nutritional Evaluation of Food Processing*. 3rd ed. New York: Van Nostrand Reinhold. Pp. 393–422.

Bone D. 1973. Water activity in intermediate moisture foods. Developing shelf-stable formulations compatible with flavor, texture, and other aspects of food is a challenge to the food technologist. *Food Technol* 27:71–76.

Brazel CS. 1999. Microencapsulation: Offering solutions for the food industry. *Cereal Food World* 44:388–396.

Briggs J, Dunn CP, Graham M, Risvik E, Cardello A, Barret A, Taub IA. 1986. *A Calorically Dense Ration for the 21st Century*. Paper presented at the 1986 Army Science Conference, West Point, NY.

Brody AL. 1989. *Controlled/Modified Atmosphere/Vacuum Packaging of Foods*. Trumbull, CT: Food & Nutrition Press.

Brody AL, Marsh KS. 1997. Foil, aluminum. In: *The Wiley Encyclopedia of Packaging Technology*. 2nd ed. New York: John Wiley & Sons. Pp. 1778–1779.

Brunauer S, Emmett PH, Teller E. 1938. Adsorption of gases in multimolecular layers. *J Am Chem Soc* 60:309–319.

Burke P. 1990. High barrier polymeric materials for increased shelf life. Activities report of the R&D Associates, Vol. 42, No. 1, San Antonio, TX.

Caldwell EF, Johnson LE, Labuza TP. 2000. Fortification and preservation of cereals. In: Fast EB, Caldwell EF, eds. *Breakfast Cereals, and How They Are Made*. 2nd ed. St. Paul, MN: American Association of Cereal Chemists. Pp. 375–410.

Cardelli C, Labuza TP. 2001. Application of Weibull Hazard Analysis to the shelf life of roasted and ground coffee. *Lebensm Wiss Technol* 34:273–278.

Cardello AV, Schutz H, Snow C, Lesher L. 2000. Predictors of food acceptance, consumption and satisfaction in specific eating situations. *Food Qual Prefer* 11:201–216.

Chinachoti P. 1998. Water migration and food storage stability. In: Taub IA, Singh RP, eds. *Food Storage Stability*. Boca Raton, FL: CRC Press. Pp. 245–268.

Corry JEL. 1978. Relationships of water activity to fungal growth. In: Beuchat LR, ed. *Food and Beverage Mycology*. Westport, CT: AVI Publishing. Pp. 45–58.

Davidsson L, Galan, P, Kastenmayer P, Cherouvrier F, Juillerat M-A, Hercberg S, Hurrell RF. 1994. Iron bioavailability studied in infants: The influence of phytic acid and ascorbic acid in infant formulas based on soy isolate. *Pediatr Res* 36:816–822.

Davidsson L, Almgren A, Hurrell RF. 1998. Sodium iron EDTA [NaFe(III)EDTA] as a food fortificant does not influence absorption and urinary excretion of manganese in healthy adults. *J Nutr* 128:1139–1143.

Davidsson L, Wzlcayk T, Zavaleta N, Hurrell R. 2001a. Improving iron absorption from a Peruvian school breakfast meal by adding ascorbic acid or $Na_2EDTA$. *Am J Clin Nutr* 73:283–287.

Davidsson L, Dimitriou T, Walczyk T, Hurrell R. 2001b. Iron absorption from experimental infant formulas based on pea (*Pisum sativum*) protein isolate: The effect of phytic acid and ascorbic acid. *Br J Nutr* 85:59–63.

Davies R, Birch GG. 1976. *Intermediate Moisture Foods*. London: Applied Science Publishers.

Deasy PB. 1984. *Microencapsulation and Related Drug Processes*. New York: Marcel Dekker.

Duyvestyen W, Shimoni E, Labuza TP. 2001. Determination of the end of shelf life for milk using Weibull Hazard Method. *Lebensm Wiss Technol* 34:143–148.

Eichner K, Karel M. 1972. The influence of water content and water activity on the sugar-amino browning reaction in model systems under various conditions. *J Agr Food Chem* 20:218–223.

Ellis B, Ripperger E, Neils Thompson J. 1961. *Design of Cushioning Systems for Air Delivery of Equipment*. Texas University Structural Research Laboratory (prepared for U.S. Army Quartermaster Research and Development Command, O.I. No. 9118, August 1961). Referenced in A Goldberg, *Foam-in-Place Concepts for Airdrop System*, Technical Report, Natick/TR-90/038L, June 1990.

Erickson LE. 1982. Recent developments in intermediate moisture foods. *J Food Protect* 45:484–491.

Fennema O, Kester JJ. 1991. Resistance of lipid films to transmission of water vapor and oxygen In: Levine H, Slade L, eds. *Water Relationships in Food: Advances in the 1980s and Trends for the 1990s*. New York: Plenum Press. Pp. 703–719.

Franks F. 1982. Water activity as a measure of biological viability and quality control. *Cereal Food World* 27:403–406.

Franks F. 1991. Hydration phenomena: An update and implications for food processing industry. In: Levine H, Slade L, eds. *Water Relationships in Foods: Advances in the 1980s and Trends for the 1990s*. New York: Plenum Press. Pp. 1–19.

Fritsch CW. 1994. Lipid oxidation—The other dimensions. *Inform* 5:423–436.

Gacula MC. 1975a. Statistical models for shelf life failures. *J Food Sci* 40:404–409.

Gacula MC. 1975b. The design of experiments for shelf life study. *J Food Sci* 40:400–403.

Gacula MC, Singh J. 1984. *Statistical Methods in Food and Consumer Research*. Orlando, FL: Academic Press.

Giese J. 2000. Shelf-life testing. *Food Technol* 54:84–85.

Goldberg A. 1990. *Foam-in-Place Concepts for Airdrop Systems*. Technical Report Natick/TR-90/038L. Natick, MA: U.S. Army Natick RD&E Center.

Gould GW. 1985. Present state of knowledge of $a_w$ effects on microorganisms. In: Simatos D, Multon JL, eds. *Properties of Water in Foods*. Dordrecht, The Netherlands: Martinus Nijhoff Publishers. Pp. 229–246.

Gregory JF III. 1996. Vitamins. In: Fennema O, ed. *Food Chemistry*. 3rd ed. New York: Marcel Dekker. Pp. 545–559.

Hallberg LM, Chinachoti P. 1992. Dynamic mechanical analysis for glass transitions in long shelf-life bread. *J Food Sci* 57:1201–1204, 1229.

Hallberg LM, Yang TCS, Taub IA. 1990. Optimization of functional ingredients in a low water activity bread using response surface methodology. In: Herz ML, Sklasrsky TA, eds. *Proceedings of the Third Natick Science Symposium*. Technical Report, Natick/TR-90/039. Natick, MA: U.S. Army Natick RD&E Center.

Han D, Yi O-S, Shin H-K. 1991. Solubilization of vitamin C in fish oil and synergistic effect with vitamin E in retarding oxidation. *J Am Oil Chem Soc* 68:740–743.

Hardas N, Danviriyakul S, Foley JL, Nawar WW, Chinachoti P. 2000. Accelerated stability studies of microencapsulated anhydrous milk fat. *Lebensm Wiss Technol* 33:506–513.

Hardas N, Danviriyakul S, Foley JL, Nawar WW, Chinachoti P. 2002. Effect of relative humidity on the oxidative and physical stability of encapsulated milk fat. *J Am Oil Chem Soc* 79:151-158.

Harper JM. 1978. Extrusion processing of food. *Food Technol* 32:67–72.

Harper JM. 1979. Food extrusion. *CRC Crit Rev Food Sci Nutr* 11:155–175.

Harper JM. 1988. Effects of extrusion processing on nutrients. In: Karmas E, Harris RS, eds. *Nutritional Evaluation of Food Processing*. 3rd ed. New York: Van Nostrand Reinhold. Pp. 365–391.

Hodge JE, Osman EM. 1976. Carbohydrates. In: Fennema OR, ed. *Principles of Food Science Part I*. New York: Marcel Dekker. Pp. 41–138.

Hurrell RF, Reddy MB, Burri J, Cook JD. 2000. An evaluation of EDTA compounds for iron fortification of cereal-based foods. *Br J Nutr* 84:903–910.

IOM (Institute of Medicine). 1993. *Nutritional Needs in Hot Environments*. Washington, DC: National Academy Press.

Jayaraman KS. 1995. Critical review on intermediate moisture fruits and vegetables. In: Barbosa-Canovas GV, Welti-Chanes J, eds. *Food Preservation by Moisture Control: Fundamentals and Applications*. Lancaster, PA: Technomic Publishing. Pp. 411–442.

Kaanane A, Labuza TP. 1989. The Maillard Reaction in foods. In: Baynes J, ed. *The Maillard Reaction in Aging, Diabetes and Nutrition*. New York: AR Liss Press. Pp 301–328.

Kaitaranta JK. 1992. Control of lipid oxidation in fish oil with various antioxidative compounds. *J Am Oil Chem Soc* 69:810–813.

Karel M. 1973. Recent research and development in the field of low-moisture and intermediate-moisture foods. *CRC Crit Rev Food Technol* 3:329–373.

Karmas E, Harris RS, eds. 1988. *Nutritional Evaluations of Food Processing*. 3rd ed. New York: Van Nostrand Reinhold.

Kirk JR. 1981. Influence of water activity on stability of vitamins in dehydrated foods. In: Rockland LB, Stewart GF, eds. *Water Activity: Influences on*

*Food Quality: A Treatise on the Influence of Bound and Free Water on the Quality and Stability of Foods and Other Natural Products*. New York: Academic Press. Pp. 531–566.

Kondo A. 1979. *Microcapsule Processing and Technology*. New York: Marcel Dekker.

Labuza TP. 1971. Kinetics of lipid oxidation in foods. *CRC Crit Rev Food Technol* 10:355–405.

Labuza TP. 1980. The effect of water activity on reaction kinetics of food deterioration. *Food Technol* 34:36–41, 59.

Labuza TP. 1982. *Shelf-Life Dating of Foods*. Westport, CT: Food & Nutrition Press.

Labuza TP. 1994. Interpreting the complexity of the kinetics of the Maillard reaction. In: Labuza TP, Reineccius GA, eds. *The Maillard Reaction in Food, Nutrition and Health*. London: Royal Society of Chemistry Press. Pp. 177–182.

Labuza TP, Saltmarch M. 1981. The non-enzymatic browning reaction as affected by water in foods. In: Rockland LB, Stewart GF, eds. *Water Activity: Influences on Food Quality: A Treatise on the Influence of Bound and Free Water on the Quality and Stability of Foods and Other Natural Products*. New York: Academic Press. Pp. 506–650.

Labuza TP, Schmidl MK. 1985. Accelerated shelf-life testing of foods. *Food Technol* 39:57–62, 64, 134.

Labuza TP, Schmidl MK. 1988. Use of sensory data in the shelf life testing of foods: Principles and graphical methods for evaluation. *Cereal Food World* 33:193–206.

Lampi RA. 1977. Flexible packaging for thermoprocessed foods. In: Mrak EM, Stewart GF, Chichester CO. *Advances in Food Research*. Vol. 23. New York: Academic Press. P. 305.

Lavoie JP, Labbe RG, Chinachoti, P. 1997. Growth of *Staphylococcus aureus* as related to $^{17}O$ NMR water mobility and water activity. *J Food Sci* 62:861–866.

Lawless HT, Heymann HG. 1999. *Sensory Evaluation of Food: Principles and Practices*. Gaithersburg, MD: Aspen Publishers. Pp. 430–475.

Lee CK. 1992. *Methods for Improved Airbag Performance for Airdrop*. Technical Report Natick/TR-93/002. Natick, MA: U.S. Army Natick RD&E Center.

Leistner L. 1995. Use of hurdle technology in food processing: Recent advances. In: Barbosa-Canovas GV, Welti-Chanes J, eds. *Food Preservation by Moisture Control: Fundamentals and Applications*. Lancaster, PA: Technomic Publishing. Pp. 377–396.

Lenovich LM. 1987. Survival and death of microorganisms as influenced by water activity. In: Rockland LB, Beuchat LR, eds. *Water Activity: Theory and Applications to Food*. New York: Marcel Dekker. Pp. 119–136.

Lin C-C, Lin S-Y, Hwang LS. 1995. Microencapsulation of squid oil with hydrophilic macromolecules for oxidative and thermal stabilization. *J Food Sci* 60:36–39.

Lindsay RC. 1996. Food additives. In: Fennema O, ed. *Food Chemistry*. 3rd ed. New York: Marcel Dekker. Pp. 780–782.

Linko P, Colona P, Mercier C. 1981. High-temperature, short-time extrusion cooking. In: Pomeranz Y, ed. *Advances in Cereal Science and Technology*. Vol. IV. St. Paul, MN: American Association of Cereal Chemists. Pp. 145–235.

Marin J, Sauer JA. 1954. *Strength of Materials*. 2nd ed. New York: MacMillan. P. 31.

Marsh KS. 1996. Food shelf-life. D-29. *Notebook Short Course May 17–19, 1997*. New Brunswick, NJ: The Center for Professional Advancement.

Meilgaard M, Civille GV, Carr BT. 1999. *Sensory Evaluation Techniques*. 3rd ed. Boca Raton, FL: CRC Press. Pp. 231–263.

Meyers MA. 1998. New encapsulated ingredients for fortified foods. Food Ingredients Europe. Conference Proceedings 1997.

Natick Research, Development, and Engineering Center. 1993. *Military specification. Bread, shelf stable, for Meal-Ready to Eat*. MIL-B-44360A. March 11, 1993. Natick, MA: Natick Research, Development, and Engineering Center.

Nawar WW. 1996. Lipids. In: Fennema O, ed. *Food Chemistry*. 3rd ed. New York: Marcel Dekker. Pp. 255–264.

Nelson KA, Labuza TP. 1992a. Relationship between water and lipid oxidation rates—Water activity and glass transition theory. In: St. Angelo AJ, ed. *Lipid Oxidation in Food*. ACS Symposium Series 500. Washington, DC: American Chemical Society.

Nelson KA, Labuza TP. 1992b. Understanding the relationship between water and lipid oxidation rates using $a_w$ and glass transition theory. In: St. Angelo M, ed. *Lipids and Food Stability*. ACS Symposium Series 500. Washington, DC: American Chemical Society. Pp. 93–103.

Nelson KA, Labuza TP. 1994. Water activity and food polymer science: Implications of state on Arrhenius and WLF models in predicting shelf life. *J Food Eng* 22:271–289.

Nielsen PV, Beuchat LR, Frisvad, JC. 1989. Influence of atmospheric oxygen content on growth and fumitremorgin production by a heat-resistant mold, *Neosartorya fischeri*. *J Food Sci* 54:679–682.

Peryam DM. 1998. Problem of preferences gets QM focus. *Food Industries* (December). In: *The 9-Point Hedonic Scale*. Peryam & Kroll Research Corporation, Chicago, IL. Pp. 1-1–1-10.

Peryam D, Girardot NF. 1952. Advanced taste-test method. *Food Eng* 24:58–61, 194.

Peryam DR, Pilgrim FJ. 1957. Hedonic scale method of measuring food preferences. *Food Technol* 11:9–14.

Pham X, Vittadini E, Levin RE, Chinachoti P. 1999. Role of water mobility on mold spore germination. *J Agric Food Chem* 47:4976–4983.

Pitt JI. 1975. Xerophilic fungi and the spoilage of foods of plant origin. In: Duckworth RB, ed. *Water Relations of Foods*. London: Academic Press. Pp. 273–308.

Pitt JI, Christian JHB. 1968. Water relations of xerophilic fungi isolated from prunes. *Appl Microbiol* 16:1853–1858.

Ponginebbi L, Nawar WW, Chinachoti P. 2000. Effect of relative humidity on lipid oxidation in freeze-dried emulsions. *Grasas y Aceites* 51:348–354.

Powers EM, Berkowitz D. 1990. Efficacy of an oxygen scavenger to modify the atmosphere and prevent mold growth on Meal, Ready-to-Eat pouch bread. *J Food Protec* 53:767–770.

Purwadaria HK, Heldman DR, Kirk JR. 1979. Computer simulation of vitamin degradation in a dry model food system during storage. *J Food Process Eng* 3:7–28.

Ragnarsson JO, Labuza TP. 1977. Accelerated shelf-life testing for oxidative rancidity in foods—A review. *Food Chem* 2:291–308.

Rahman MS, Labuza TP. 1999. Water activity and food preservation. In: Rahman MS, ed. *Handbook of Food Preservation*. New York: Marcel Dekker. Pp. 339–382.

Reid DS. 1995. Chemical reactivity as a function of solutes with particular reference to carbohydrate. In: Barbosa-Canovas GV, Welti-Chanes J, eds. *Food Preservation by Moisture Control: Fundamentals and Applications*. Lancaster, PA: Technomic Publishing. Pp. 227–253.

Risch SJ, Reineccius GA, eds. 1995. *Encapsulation and Controlled Release of Food Ingredients*. ACS Symposium Series No. 590. Washington, DC: American Chemical Society.

Riordan P. 1970. *Weather Extremes Around the World*. Technical Report 70-45-E5. Natick, MA: U.S. Army Natick Laboratories.

Roos JG. 1993. Hitting the mark in Bosnia. *Armed Forces J Int* June:58.

Roos Y, Karel M. 1991. Water and molecular weight effects on glass transitions in amorphous carbohydrates and carbohydrate solutions. *J Food Sci* 56:1676 1681.

Rossen JL, Miller RC. 1973. Food extrusion. *Food Technol* 27:46–53.

Ruan RR, Chen PL. 1998. *Water in Foods and Biological Materials: A Nuclear Magnetic Resonance Approach*. Lancaster, PA: Technomic Publishing. Pp. 149–228.

Salame M. 1974. The use of low permeation thermoplastics in food and beverage packaging. In: Hopdenberg HB, Stannett V eds. *Permeability of Plastic Films and Coatings to Gases, Vapors, and Liquids (Proceeding of the Borden Award Symposium of the Division of Organic Coatings and*

*Plastics Chemistry of the American Chemical Society, honoring Professor Vivian T. Stannett).* New York: Plenum Publishing. P. 275.

Saltmarch M, Labuza TP. 1982. Nonenzymatic browning via the Maillard reaction in foods. *Diabetes* 31:29–36.

Salunkhe DK, Wu MT, Do JY. 1979. Effects of long-term storage on quality of processed foods. I. Meal, Ready-To-Eat, Individual ration items packed in flexible retortable pouches. *J Food Quality* 2:75–103.

Saroka W. 1999. *Fundamentals of Packaging Technology.* Herndon, VA: Institute of Packaging Professionals.

SBCOMM (U.S. Army Soldier and Biological Chemical Command). 2001a. Food Packet, Survival, General Purpose (GP). Fact Sheet. Natick, MA: Soldier Systems Center.

SBCOMM. 2001b. Meal, Ready-to-Eat, Individual (MRE). Fact Sheet. Natick, MA: Soldier Systems Center.

Schulz GL, Meyer A, Taub I, Berkowitz D, Cardello A, Hirsch E, Dunne CP, Narayan A, Atwood B, Porter W, Silverman G. 1992. Military Food. In: Hui Y-H, ed. *Encyclopedia of Food Science and Technology.* Vol. 3. New York: John Wiley & Sons. Pp. 1778–1789.

Shimada Y, Roos Y, Karel M. 1991. Oxidation of methyl linoleate encapsulated in amorphous lactose-based food model. *J Agr Food Chem* 39:637–641.

Slade L, Levine H. 1991. A food polymer science approach to structure-property relationships in aqueous food systems: Non-equilbrium behavior of carbohydrate-water systems. In: Levine H, Slade L, eds. *Water Relationships in Foods: Advances in the 1980s and Trends for the 1990s.* New York: Plenum Press. Pp. 29–101.

Sloan AE, Waletzko PT, Labuza TP. 1976. Effect of order-of-mixing on $a_w$ lowering ability of food humectants. *J Food Sci* 41:536–540.

Smith OB. 1982. Extrusion cooking of corn flours and starches as snacks, breadings, croutons, breakfast cereals, pastas, food thickeners, and adhesives. In: Inglett GE, ed. *Maize, Recent Progress in Chemistry and Technology.* New York: Academic Press. Pp. 193–220.

Stone H, Sidel JL. 1993. *Sensory Evaluation Practices.* 2nd ed. San Diego: Academic Press. Pp. 243–270.

Szczeblowski JW. 1971. *An Assessment of the Flexible Packaging System for Heat Processed Foods.* Technical Report 71-57-GP. Natick, MA: U.S. Army Natick Laboratories.

Taoukis P, Breene W, Labuza TP. 1988. Intermediate moisture foods. In: Pomeranz Y, ed. *Advances in Cereal Science and Technology.* Vol. IX. St. Paul, MN: American Association of Cereal Chemists. Pp. 91–128.

Troller JA. 1987. Adaptation and growth of microorganisms in environments with reduced water activity. In: Rockland LB, Beuchat LR, eds. *Water Activity: Theory and Applications to Food.* New York: Marcel Dekker. Pp. 101–117.

Troller JA, Christian JHB. 1978. Microbial growth. In: Troller JA, Christian JHB eds. *Water Activity and Food.* New York: Academic Press. Pp. 86–102.

Vaamonde G, Cherife J, Scorza OC. 1982. An examination of minimal water activity for *Staphylococcus aureus* ATCC 6538 P growth in laboratory media adjusted with less conventional solutes. *J Food Sci* 47:1259–1262.

Van Campen DR, Glahn RP. 1999. Micronutrient bioavailability techniques: Accuracy, problems and limitations. *Field Crop Res* 60:93–113.

Velasco J, Dobarganes MC, Marquez-Ruiz G. 2000. Oxidation of free and encapsulated oil fractions in dried microencapsulated fish oils. *Grasas Aceites* 51:439–446.

Villota R, Hawkes JG. 1992. Reaction kinetics in food systems. In: Heldman DR, Lund DB, eds. *Handbook of Food Engineering*. New York: Marcel Dekker. Pp. 39–144.

Warmbier HC, Schnickels RA, Labuza TP. 1976. Effect of glycerol on nonenzymatic browning in a solid intermediate moisture model food system. *J Food Sci* 41:528–531.

Young H, Fellows P, Mitchell J. 1985. Development of a high energy biscuit for use as a food supplement in disaster relief. *J Food Technol* 20:689–695.

# 4

# Performance Specifications

## ITEM DESCRIPTION

This product—the high-energy, nutrient-dense emergency relief food product (EFP)—is intended to provide a compact, self-contained, high-energy, nutrient-dense emergency food for refugees and victims of disasters for a short duration at the initial stages of an emergency. The expected use period is 3 to 7 days, with a maximum use of up to 15 days. The product may be used in climatic extremes from arctic to tropical. The EFP is expected to be the sole source of food during the period of use and to provide adequate energy, protein, fat, vitamins, and minerals to promote survivability. The product may be consumed directly or crumbled to make a gruel or porridge.

The EFP must be suitable for a wide age range—from infants over 6 months through older adults.

The EFP must be provided in a format acceptable to people from a wide range of ethnic, cultural, and religious backgrounds.

The EFP will be consumed under worldwide environmental extremes. It is essential that this item be produced in accordance with Good Manufacturing Practices applicable to ready-to-eat food products.

There are five characteristics critical to development of a successful EFP. These are listed in order of importance. The EFP must be:

1. Safe
2. Palatable
3. Easy to dispense
4. Easy to use
5. Nutritionally complete.

## PERFORMANCE REQUIREMENTS

### Nutrition

The EFP must provide a nutritional profile as described in Table 4-1. Each unit (nine bars) will provide 2,100 kcal.

### Shelf Life

The packaged EFP shall meet the minimum shelf-life requirement of 36 months at 21° C (70° F).

### Appearance

1. **Exterior** – The EFP will be a bar of a rectangular shape that promotes efficient packing. The color of the bar will depend on the ingredients and processing methods used. Artificial colors are not recommended, and it is required that the product not be white or cream-colored. The product, if dispersed in water, must not resemble milk.
2. **Interior** – The EFP shall be a compressed, cold-extruded, or baked product of essentially uniform composition.
3. **General** – The packaged EFP shall be free from foreign material such as, but not limited to, dirt, insect parts, hair, wood, glass, or metal. The product shall show no evidence of excessive heating (materially darkened or scorched).

### Odor and Flavor

1. The EFP shall be slightly sweet with blended cereal flavor from the base ingredients, and no distinct flavor notes attributable to the protein source or vitamin and mineral additions may be present. Flavorings may be used, but should not be strong or unusual (i.e., not targeted for a specific population).
2. The EFP shall be free from foreign odors and flavors such as, but not limited to, burnt, scorched, rancid, sour, or stale.

### Texture

The texture of the bars will depend on the ingredients and processing methods used. When crumbled, particle size should be large enough to make a porridge-like product when dispersed in water, and not small enough to resemble milk. The EFP shall be sufficiently firm and resilient to withstand delivery via various modes of transportation (air, land, and sea) including low-altitude airdrop. It must maintain structural integrity through short periods of extreme temperatures.

## Size

The EFP dimensions shall be such that a unit will deliver 2,100 kcal and be divided into nine bars, each bar scored to yield two equal portions. Each portion will contain approximately 116 kcal. The total net weight of the unit (2,100 kcal/EFP) shall be approximately 450 g (~50 g/EFP bar).

## Acceptability

A prototype of the finished product shall be tested by the procuring agency and must receive a hedonic score of 6.0 or better on a 1.0- to 9.0-point scale, where 9.0 represents "like extremely" when assessed by likely target populations under conditions simulating field use (e.g., during 3 to 7 days' consumption).

## Nutrient Content

The nutrient content is described in Table 4-1. The overall description is:

- **Energy content** – The EFP shall be designed as a 2,100-kcal unit.
- **Moisture content** – The moisture content shall not be greater than 9.5 percent. Water activity shall not be greater than 0.6.
- **Protein content** – The protein content shall be not less than 63 or greater than 80 g/2,100-kcal unit (8 to 9 g/EFP bar). The protein must have a minimum Protein Digestibility-Corrected Amino Acid Score of 1.0.
- **Lipids** – The lipids must be 22 percent by weight minimum (approximately 40 percent of kcal, 82 to 105 g/2,100 kcal unit, or 9 to 12 g/EFP bar). The source of lipids must not be lard, tallow, other animal fats, or similar animal-based products. The ratio of linoleic acid to α-linolenic acid shall be 5:1 to 10:1.
- **Carbohydrates** – The remaining calories will come from carbohydrates as specified in Table 4-1.
- **Vitamins and minerals** – As specified in Table 4-1.

Note: Vitamin E must be encapsulated (or stabilized) for stability. Separate encapsulation is also necessary for ascorbic acid and for metals: iron (as NaFe EDTA), chromium, copper, manganese, selenium, and zinc.

- **Caloric density** must be between 233 and 250 kcal/50 g bar (2,100 kcal/unit).

## Additives

Additives must be consistent with guidelines of both the U.S. Food and Drug Administration (FDA) and Codex Alimentarius, and comply with the

**TABLE 4-1** Nutrient Specifications for a High-Energy, Nutrient-Dense, Emergency Relief Food Product (EFP)[a]

| Nutrient | Minimum Required Nutrient Density/EFP Bar (50 g) | Maximum Required Nutrient Density/EFP Bar (50 g) | Minimum Required Nutrient Density/1,000 kcal |
|---|---|---|---|
| Energy | 233 kcal | 250 kcal | |
| Fat | 9.1 g (35% of calories) | 11.7 g (45% of calories) | 39 g (35% of calories) |
| Protein[b] | 7.9 g (13.5% of calories) | 8.9 g (15% of calories) | 34 g (13.5% of calories) |
| Total carbohydrates | | | 100–125 g (40–50% of calories) |
| Total sugars | 7–11.7 g (12–20% of calories) | 14.7 g (25% of calories) | 30–50 g (12–20% of calories) |
| Glucose | 2 g | | 8.5 g |
| Lactose | | 4 g | |
| Monosaccharides | | 5.8 g | |
| Sodium | 0.30 g | 0.33 g | 1.3 g |
| Potassium | 0.40 g | 0.47 g | 1.7 g |
| Chloride | 0.47 g | 0.51 g | 2.0 g |
| Calcium | 180 mg | 207 mg | 768 mg |
| Phosphorus | 172 mg | 206 mg | 740 mg |
| Magnesium | 44 mg | 54 mg | 190 mg |
| Chromium | 3.0 μg | | 13 μg |
| Copper | 131 μg | 156 μg | 560 μg |
| Iodine | 24.5 μg | 53.6 μg | 105 μg |

| Maximum Allowed Nutrient Density/1,000 kcal | Minimum Required Nutrient Density/2,100 kcal | Maximum Allowed Nutrient Density/2,100 kcal | Comments |
|---|---|---|---|
| | 2,100 kcal | | 2,100–2,250 kcal/9 bars |
| 50 g (45% of calories) | 82 g (35% of calories) | 105 g (45% of calories) | Saturated fat > 10% of calories; PUFA 7–10% of calories from vegetable oil; LA:LNA ratio of 5:1 to 10:1 |
| 38 g (15% of calories) | 71 g (13.5% of calories) | 80 g (15% of calories) | PDCAAS ≥ 1.00 |
| | 210–263 g | | |
| 63 g (25% of calories) | 63–105 g (12–20% of calories) | 131 g (25% of calories) | Palatability requires the use of sugar or high fructose corn syrup |
| | 18 g | | 6 g/g of Na; from maltodextrins |
| 17 g | | 36 g | Should be present only if milk solids are used |
| 25 g | | 53 g | < 25% by weight of carbohydrates |
| 1.4 g | 2.7 g | 3.0 g | EFP should not taste salty |
| 2.0 g | 3.5 g | 4.2 g | EFP should not taste bitter |
| 2.2 g | 4.2 g | 4.6 g | Equimolar to sodium |
| 885 mg | 1,620 mg | 1,865 mg | Phosphate, citrate, or carbonate salt forms |
| 890 mg | 1,555 mg | 1,865 mg | Nonphytate form |
| 230 mg (< 167 mg as supplement) | 400 mg | 480 mg (< 350 mg as supplement) | Only supplemental Mg contributes to UL |
| | 27 μg | | |
| 670 μg | 1,180 μg | 1,410 μg | |
| 230 μg | 220 μg | 480 μg | |

*continued*

**TABLE 4-1** Continued

| Nutrient | Minimum Required Nutrient Density/EFP Bar (50 g) | Maximum Required Nutrient Density/EFP Bar (50 g) | Minimum Required Nutrient Density/1,000 kcal |
|---|---|---|---|
| Iron[c] | 3.7 mg | 4.2 mg | 16 mg |
| Manganese | 0.33 mg | 0.40 mg | 1.4 mg |
| Selenium | 6.5 µg | 7.9 µg | 28 µg |
| Zinc | 2.4 mg | 2.7 mg | 10.4 mg |
| Vitamin A (preformed) | 117 µg | 233 µg | 500 µg |
| Vitamin D | 1.2 µg | 1.4 µg | 5.2 µg |
| Vitamin E | 2.2 mg | | 16 mg |
| Vitamin K | 14 µg | | 60 µg |
| Vitamin C | 23.3 mg | 46.6 mg | 100 mg |
| Thiamin | 0.28 mg | 0.33 mg | 1.2 mg |
| Riboflavin | 0.28 mg | 0.33 mg | 1.2 mg |
| Niacin | 2.6 mg | 2.9 mg | 11.2 mg |
| Vitamin $B_6$ | 0.28 mg | 0.33 mg | 1.2 mg |
| Folate[d] | 45.2 µg | 49.7 µg | 194 µg |
| Vitamin $B_{12}$ | 2.8 µg | 3.4 µg | 12 µg |
| Pantothenic Acid | 0.9 mg | 1.1 mg | 3.9 mg |
| Biotin | 5.6 µg | 6.7 µg | 24 µg |
| Choline | 85.3 mg | 102.3 mg | 366 mg |

[a] The energy content of the EFP is specified as 4.5 to 5 kcal/g, which provides a range of 2,100 to 2,250 kcal per 9-bar ration (EFP). It is important to note that calculation of nutrient density for all other nutrients is based on the minimum energy requirement for the EFP of 2,100 kcal (IOM, 1995). Calculations based on information in the text may differ slightly from the numbers presented in the table due to rounding.

[b] Protein digestibility-corrected amino acid score (PDCAAS) is a method described by FAO/WHO (1989) for protein evaluation that is based on the essential amino acid requirements of the 2- to 5-year-old child. The use of this method of protein evaluation by U.S. food manufacturers has Food and Drug Administration approval.

| Maximum Allowed Nutrient Density/1,000 kcal | Minimum Required Nutrient Density/2,100 kcal | Maximum Allowed Nutrient Density/2,100 kcal | Comments |
|---|---|---|---|
| 18 mg | 34 mg | 38 mg | Encapsulated as NaFeEDTA suggested |
| 1.7 mg | 2.9 mg | 3.5 mg | |
| 34 μg | 60 μg | 72 μg | Selenomethionine form |
| 11.4 mg | 22 mg | 24 mg | Sulfate or acetate; molar ratio of Zn:phytate < 15 |
| 1,000 μg | 1,050 μg | 2,100 μg | Does not include carotene |
| 5.8 μg | 11 μg | 12 μg | Cholecalciferol form |
| | 34 mg | | 0.6 mg/g PUFA |
| | 120 μg | | |
| 200 mg | 210 mg | 420 mg | Encapsulation required |
| 1.4 mg | 2.5 mg | 3.0 mg | |
| 1.4 mg | 2.5 mg | 3.0 mg | |
| 12.4 mg | 23.6 mg | 26.0 mg | Maximum only refers to added nicotinic acid |
| 1.4 mg | 2.5 mg | 3.0 mg | |
| 213 μg | 406 μg | 447 μg | Maximum only refers to added folate |
| 14.4 μg | 25.2 μg | 30.2 μg | |
| 4.7 mg | 8.2 mg | 9.8 mg | |
| 28.8 μg | 50.4 μg | 60.5 μg | |
| 439 mg | 769 mg | 923 mg | Choline could be provided as lecithin |

[c] Iron requirements based on FAO/WHO (2000) for adolescent girls, which assumes 10% bioavailability.

[d] Assumes that folate provided will be as a food fortificant and thus will be synthetic folate, which is 1.6 times more available than naturally occurring food folate.

specifications set forth in the Food Chemicals Codex (National Academy Press, Washington, D.C.).

## PROHIBITIONS

The EFP shall contain no sensitive ingredients that would limit its intended use for diverse populations. No alcohol shall be incorporated in it, nor any meat products used.

## PROCESSING REQUIREMENTS

Bars shall be prepared through extrusion, compression technology, or baked.

Units will be prepared consisting of nine bars of approximately 233 kcal each, with central scores that allow easy division to 116-kcal portions.

It is desirable that the EFP be amenable to being made into a gruel by crumbling the bar and mixing with water.

## PACKAGING REQUIREMENTS

The EFP will be subjected to environments that exhibit a wide range, including extremes, of temperature and humidity, and to delivery conditions that will often be characterized by lack of infrastructure. Therefore, all packaging components must be capable of withstanding temperature and physical abuse. In addition, the EFP will be delivered using all modes of transportation, including airdrop. Separate packaging, or more likely, additional packaging, may be employed for airdrop requirements.

### Primary Packaging

Each 2,100-kcal daily EFP unit will be prepared as nine equal-sized bars, each centrally scored to allow breaking into two segments. The nine bars will be individually wrapped to facilitate handling of individual bars, while reducing contamination to additional bars, through human, insect, animal, or microbial intervention. The primary wrap need not be a barrier material, and it is recommended that it be pulp-based, with a moisture-barrier coating. The coating may be polyolefin or wax-based. This primary package, after use, may also serve as an energy source through combustion. Polyethylene- or wax-coated paper both provide similar heating value as comparable weights of fuel oils. The package will be nitrogen flushed. Residual oxygen must not exceed 3 percent (2 percent if feasible).

## Secondary Packaging

A daily supply of nine bars will be packaged under a nitrogen flush or a vacuum, into a barrier package, to enhance product shelf life. The secondary packaging will be a pouch construction similar to the trilaminate construction utilized by the military for long shelf-life rations: from inside to outside, 0.003- to 0.004-in thick polyolefin, 0.00035- to 0.0007-in thick aluminum foil, and 0.0005-in thick polyester or nylon. The pouch material shall be FDA-approved for food use and shall show no evidence of delamination or degradation when heat sealed or fabricated into pouches. Pouches that contain the nine bars may be preformed or formed on line. The pouches will have an inside dimension sufficient to hold the nine individually wrapped bars. The pouch shall be made by heat-sealing three edges (two sides and bottom) with 3/8-in- (+/- 1/8 in) wide seals. The heat seals shall be made in a manner that will ensure hermetic seals. The pouch shall maintain its integrity and air tightness of the side and bottom seals when tested by appropriate methods. The side and bottom seals shall have an average seal strength of not less than 6.0 lb/in, and no individual specimen shall have a seal strength of less than 5.0 lb/in. A V-, C-, or U-shaped tear notch at least 1/32-in deep, located 3/4 to 1 in from the top edge of the pouch (excluding the lip) shall be made on one or both side seals. The distance between the inside edge of the tear notch and the inside edge of the seal shall be no less than 1/8 in. One side of the open end of the pouch may be provided with an extended or fold-over lip, extended not more than 1/8 in (+/- 1/16 in) to facilitate opening and filling. In order to discourage diversion of the product, the pouch must be of a neutral color (e.g., off-white, tan); no bright, attractive colors or shine may be used.

A multiple set of bars, sufficient for a 5-day supply of nine bars per day (i.e., five pouches containing nine bars each) will be packaged together and constitute the distribution unit called a "bundle." The five trilaminate pouches will be bundled into a low-density polyethylene bag to provide either a 5-day individual EFP supply or a daily ration for a family of five members. The film used to prepare the bundle will be monoaxially or biaxially oriented, with machine direction oriented across the pouch. Filling will therefore be accomplished on a horizontal wrapping machine. A V-, C-, or U-shaped tear notch at least 1/32-in deep, located 3/4 to 1 in from the top edge of the pouch (excluding the lip) shall be made on one or both side seals. The notch will allow easy opening by propagating the notch tear across the bundle bag.

As an alternative, the outer package may be a reusable, semi-rigid polyolefin container which could be used for storage and/or water transport.

A third option is to utilize a metal outer package, such as a tinplate box with a cover. The cover shall be easily removable. This container may also have multiple uses, such as storage and/or water carrier.

### Tertiary Packaging

Rations will be available in two formats: Ground delivery and airdrop.

- **Ground delivery** – Eight bundles consisting of five pouches each (each pouch contains five daily units) will be placed in a 4×2 configuration in a corrugated shipping container that constitutes 1 case. Approximately 50 cases will be placed on a pallet. The shipper will be sufficient to contain the rations and allow stacking to five pallets high in similar environmental temperature and relative humidity extremes as experienced in the Guam, Italy, and Maryland storage facilities used by the U.S. Agency for International Development.
- **Airdrop** – Pouches (five units each) or bundles (five pouches each) may be packaged for low-altitude airdrop using appropriate package protection to simultaneously provide impact protection for the EFP and reduce the terminal velocity to a level that prevents injury to recipients on the ground. Testing must be conducted to verify adequate protection.

### Labeling

The secondary and tertiary packaging shall carry simple, graphic instructions on how to open the package and on alternative ways to consume the product (i.e., directly or as a porridge). A disclosure of the energy nutrient (fat, carbohydrate, protein) content by weight, in metric units, must be made on the basis of 1 day's ration (2,100 kcal). In addition, each pouch shall carry a complete list of ingredients, the net weight of the unit, in grams, and any other information required by the purchasing agency.

## MISCELLANEOUS INFORMATION

Ingredients may be determined by bid from potential manufacturers to provide the nutritional profile and other characteristics defined above. The product will be distributed among multiple ethnic and cultural groups. Therefore, alcohol or animal products other than milk may not be used. Foods containing known allergens, such as peanuts, should be avoided.

The vitamin and mineral mix must be encapsulated to provide required product shelf life and avoid objectionable odors or flavors.

Recommended ingredients:

- **Cereal base**: wheat flour, corn, oat flakes or flour, rice flour
- **Protein**: soy products, such as concentrates, isolates, or TVP; milk solids, casein, or derivatives
- **Lipid sources**: partially hydrogenated soybean or cottonseed oil, flaxseed oil (source of omega-3 fatty acids), canola oil, sunflower oil
- **Sugars**: sucrose, glucose, high-fructose corn syrup, maltodextrins

- **Baking and leavening agents**, if needed
- **Vitamin and mineral premix** as specified in the nutrient profile (see Table 4-1).

The product must be prepared using Good Manufacturing Practices and maintain suitability as a food for the shelf life of the product.

Note: This performance specification is written to facilitate innovation from suppliers. It is recommended that off-the-shelf ingredients and materials be utilized where possible.

# Appendix

# Biographical Sketches of Subcommittee Members

**Barry L. Zoumas, Ph.D.** (*chair*) is the Alan R. Warehime Professor of Agribusiness in the Department of Agricultural Economics and Rural Sociology at The Pennsylvania State University. Dr. Zoumas' academic training is in human nutrition and chemistry. He has direct expertise in development of the type of food product under study. He was Director of Research and Development and later Corporate Vice-President of science and technology at Hershey Foods Corporation, where he was in charge of development of the Hershey bars for the space program before joining Penn State. He is coauthor of a book on candy bars. He also has ample international experience as a visiting scientist in nutrition programs for developing countries with the Food and Agriculture Organization of the United Nations and as an advisor on agricultural development to the U.S. Agency for International Development for the Caribbean and other Latin American countries. He has served as Chairman of the American Institute of Nutrition and several industrial associations, and is a member of the Institute of Food Technologists, the American Association for the Advancement of Science, the American Chemical Society, the American Society for Nutritional Sciences, and the International Food and Agribusiness Management Association.

**Lawrence E. Armstrong, Ph.D.** is an Associate Professor in the Departments of Physiology, Neurobiology and Exercise Science and of Sport, Leisure, and Exercise Sciences, University of Connecticut. He has a doctorate in human bioenergetics and specializes in physiological responses involving exercise, dietary intervention, heat tolerance, temperature regulation, and acclimatization to heat. His research deals with laboratory and field studies of metabolic, ventilatory, cardiovascular, fluid-electrolyte, and strength perturbations, viewed in light of physical training, cardiorespiratory fitness, and hydration status. He teaches courses in exercise physiology and metabolism. Dr. Armstrong is a former member of the Committee on Military Nutrition Research. He is also a member of the American College of Sports Medicine, American Physiological Society, and the Aerospace Medical Association.

**Jeffrey R. Backstrand, Ph.D.** is an Associate Professor in the joint Ph.D. Program on Urban Systems at the University of Medicine and Dentistry of New Jersey. Previous to this position he was Assistant Professor and Director of the Public Health Nutrition Program at the New York University Department of Nutrition and Food Studies. His academic training is in nutritional anthropology. His research interests are sociocultural determinants of food intake and food sources of micronutrients in developing countries. He has conducted research and has supervised several Ph.D. dissertations and M.S. theses dealing with various aspects of food preferences in Korea, Niger, and Mexico. He has written papers on fortification and growth in children in developing countries, with an emphasis on Mexico. He is Chair of the Public Nutrition Research Interest Section, American Society for Nutritional Sciences and a fellow of the Society for Applied Anthropology. He is also a member of the American Anthropological Association, the American Public Health Association, the Association for the Study of Food and Society, and the Council on Nutritional Anthropology

**Wanda L. Chenoweth, Ph.D.** is Professor of Nutritional Sciences in the Department of Food Science and Human Nutrition, Michigan State University. Her area of expertise is clinical dietetics, and her research interests are in mineral bioavailability and clinical nutrition. She has conducted research also on the effects of processing on the nutritional quality of various food ingredients. Dr. Chenoweth is a member of the American Society for Nutritional Sciences, American Dietetic Association, and the Institute of Food Technologists. She is a member of the Committee on Military Nutrition Research.

**Pavinee Chinachoti, Ph.D.** is Professor of Food Physico-chemistry, Department of Food Science and Nutrition, University of Massachusetts, Amherst. Dr. Chinachoti teaches food processing at the graduate and undergraduate levels. Her research focuses on characterization of phase transitions and the role of water on food quality and stability, particularly in cereal polymers and products. It includes staling mechanisms, moisture migration, recrystallization of sugars and other carbohydrates, and water activity in relation to microbial spoilage and pathogenic microorganisms, applied to various foods and intermediate moisture foods. She has conducted joint research with the U. S. Army Natick technical group and is a member of the Institute of Food Technologists, Sigma Xi Scientific Research Society, Gamma Sigma Delta Agricultural Honorary Society, Phi Kappa Phi Honorary Society, and Phi Tau Sigma Honorary Society.

**Barbara P. Klein, Ph.D.** is Emeritus Professor of Foods and Nutrition in the Department of Food Science and Human Nutrition, University of Illinois. Her areas of expertise are sensory perception and evaluation and development of high soy protein foods such as snacks, cereals, and dairy analogs. Her research is in the areas of formula and sensory optimization of food products manufactured with high protein ingredients, vitamin C content of various foods, nutrient conservation in processed food products, sensory science in general, and in alterations in food quality that occur during storage, processing, and preparation for consumption. Dr. Klein is a member of the Institute of Food Technologists, American Institute of Nutrition, American Chemical Society, American Dietetic Association, and American Society for Testing Materials.

**Helen W. Lane, Ph.D., R.D.** is Chief Nutritionist and Program Manager for Advanced Human Support Technology at the NASA Johnson Space Center. Dr. Lane has extensive experience on the relationship of diet and exercise and on diet formulation. Her research has focused on nutritional aspects of space flight, nutrient availability, body composition, and nutritional requirements for energy, water, electrolytes, protein, calcium, and iron. Her work as NASA's Advanced Human Support Technologies Program includes innovative work in food science and technologies for extended-duration space flight. She is a member of numerous societies, among them the American Dietetic Association, American Society for Nutritional Sciences, American Society of Clinical Nutrition, Institute of Food Technologists, and Sigma Xi Scientific Research Society.

**Kenneth S. Marsh, Ph.D.** is President/Research Director of Kenneth S. Marsh & Associates, Ltd. While with the Packaging Science Department at Clemson University, Dr. Marsh held the CRYOVAC Chair, the first endowed position in Packaging Science in the United States. Dr. Marsh's academic background is in food science, with specialization in food packaging. His research focuses on utilizing physical chemistry, food science, and packaging to extend the useable life of foods, reduce distribution damage, and improve the deliverable food supply in poor countries. He has 12 years of food industry experience (Quaker Oats Company, Ball Corporation, Pillsbury Company, and Thomas J. Lipton, Inc.), and 16 years of experience as a private consultant in food packaging. Dr. Marsh also has had extensive international exposure as a lecturer in various aspects of food packaging and has participated in packaging-related activities of Research & Development Associates. He is a member of the Institute of Food Technologists and the Institute of Packaging Professionals, and is a Fellow of the Institute of Packaging Professionals

**Marjatta Tolvanen, Ph.D.** is Project Officer in Nutrition in Emergencies with the United Nations Children's Fund, New York. She is an international nutritionist from Finland in charge of monitoring nutritional emergencies in various countries and coordinating emergency responses. Dr. Tolvanen also conducts assessments of the impact of using special feeding products for emergency feeding and oversees development of such products for UNICEF. She has international experience in Vietnam and Nepal.